The Brain Explained

Alex Rossi

Copyright © 2024 Alex Rossi

All rights reserved.

ISBN: 9798337655406

CONTENTS

1 The Anatomy of the Brain .... Pg 7

2 Neurochemistry and Neurotransmitters .... Pg 23

3 Cognitive Functions .... Pg 38

4 Emotions and the Brain .... Pg 53

5 Sensory and Motor Pathways .... Pg 72

6 The Developing Brain .... Pg 91

7 Brain Disorders and Diseases .... Pg 107

8 The Future of Brain Research .... Pg 124

INTRODUCTION

Welcome to "The Brain Explained," a comprehensive guide designed to demystify the intricate world of the brain. This book is your journey through the labyrinthine pathways of the human brain, exploring each fold and fissure from A to Z. Geared to peel back the layers of complexity surrounding the brain's function and structure, it aims to make the science accessible, engaging, and thoroughly understandable.

I want to apologize that there are no illustrations in this book, so it may be handy to have a laptop or a tablet open to view certain parts of the brain that we discuss for a better illustration.

Our brains, the command centers of our bodies, are endlessly fascinating. They hold the keys to our thoughts, memories, emotions, and intricate motor functions, managing everything from our breathing patterns to our most complex critical thinking tasks. However, despite its central role in our existence, the brain remains one of the most enigmatic and misunderstood organs in the human body.

In "The Brain Explained," we break down the brain's anatomy and functionality into digestible sections, each dedicated to a different aspect of this remarkable organ. Whether you're curious about the cerebral cortex, mesmerized by the mysteries of memory, or seeking clarity on the nervous system, this book translates intricate neuroscience into simple language. Alongside clear explanations are vivid examples and relatable analogies that bring the dry and often complex topics to life, making the content not only more understandable but also more relatable.

Prepare to embark on a narrative journey that integrates current theories about the brain with tangible, real-world applications and insights. From the basics of neuron functions to advanced topics like neuroplasticity and cognitive decline, "The Brain Explained" offers a panoramic view into the cerebral universe that resides within each of us.

Readers can expect to emerge with a more nuanced understanding of how the brain operates, the factors that affect its health, and the future possibilities that current research might yield. This book is not just an educational resource; it is an invitation to become more aware of the incredibly sophisticated organ that influences every aspect of human life.

"The Brain Explained" is an essential read for anyone looking to deepen their knowledge of the brain, providing the tools to better understand oneself and the neural workings that influence our daily existence. With every page, you'll be closer to mastering the fundamentals of the brain, empowered by knowledge that was, until now, veiled in academic mystery. Welcome to a clearer understanding of your brain.

THE ANATOMY OF THE BRAIN

The brain, a marvel of biological engineering, is at the core of everything we do, think, and perceive. It's here where thoughts form, memories weave together, and emotions ebb and flow—a result of complex neural interactions. Understanding its structure—the cerebrum, cerebellum, and brainstem—is not just about charting parts but appreciating how seamlessly they function together to manage our daily lives. These regions, although distinct, work in unison like a well-conducted orchestra, ensuring our bodies respond appropriately to constant internal and external changes. This intricate interplay governs not only basic survival processes but also our highest forms of cognition and coordination. By exploring the anatomy of the brain, we reveal the underpinnings of human behavior and the physiological processes that support our most sophisticated mental functions. This knowledge equips us with a deeper understanding of our own actions and experiences, illustrated through the brain's remarkable capacity to process and respond to complex information.

The cerebrum stands as the largest part of the human brain and is pivotal for cognitive functions such as thinking, memory, and decision-making. Encased in the skull, the cerebrum is divided into two hemispheres, each responsible for different yet interconnected tasks. The right hemisphere excels in visual and spatial tasks, aiding in artistic endeavors and recognition of patterns, while the left hemisphere is crucial for language, reasoning, and analytical thinking.

Each hemisphere is further divided into lobes, each overseeing specific mental and physical functions. The frontal lobes, located at the front of the brain, play a critical role in advanced cognitive processes such as planning, forming ideas, making decisions, and moderating social behavior. They are similar to the CEO of a company, making high-level decisions that affect the entire body.

Behind the frontal lobes lie the parietal lobes, essential for integrating sensory information from various parts of the body, understanding numbers, and manipulating objects. When you navigate through a crowded room or knead dough to bake bread, your parietal lobes are at work, processing textures and spatial relationships.

The occipital lobes, situated at the back of the brain, are primarily involved in visual processing. Whenever you read a book or admire a sunset, these lobes are activating, translating photons into coherent images.

Lastly, the temporal lobes, located on each side of the brain, are pivotal for processing auditory information and are crucial in the formation of memories. When recalling a piece of music or a conversation from earlier in the day, your temporal lobes are engaging.

While each lobe's functionality is distinct, the cerebrum is not a series of isolated units but a deeply interconnected network where seamless communication is constant. This communication is facilitated by millions of neurons, connected by synapses that transmit electrochemical signals swiftly and efficiently. This network's functionality is crucial for transforming real-time sensory data into coherent, thoughtful actions and reactions.

Understanding the architecture and functionality of the cerebrum not only sheds light on how we perform everyday activities but also highlights the complexity and elegance of the human brain. This awareness bridges the gap between abstract neurological concepts and tangible, everyday experiences, illustrating how deeply our brain's structure influences our daily lives and overall human capacity.

The cerebral cortex, the brain's outermost layer, is intricately divided into four primary lobes: the frontal, parietal, occipital, and temporal. Each lobe hosts distinct cognitive and physical functions, facilitated by specialized neurons and neurotransmitters, interacting seamlessly with one another and the broader nervous system.

The **frontal lobes** are key players in executive functions, including decision-making, problem-solving, and controlling social behavior. They house pyramidal neurons, which are crucial for voluntary movement and cognitive functions because of their long axons that transmit signals over great distances within the brain. Dopamine, a neurotransmitter linked to reward and attention mechanisms, has a significant presence here, influencing both motivation and focus.

In the **parietal lobes**, sensory information from the body is processed, aiding in spatial orientation and movement coordination. These lobes are rich in somatosensory neurons, which process signals related to touch, pressure, and pain. The neurotransmitter acetylcholine is prevalent, playing a vital role in learning and memory by enhancing sensory perception and attention.

The **occipital lobes** are primarily concerned with visual processing. They contain a high density of neurons responsible for interpreting visual stimuli, including colors, motion, and shapes. The neurotransmitter glutamate is abundant here, facilitating fast signal transmission essential for the rapid processing speeds required for visual recognition.

The **temporal lobes** manage auditory information and are integral to memory formation. They feature a variety of neuron types, including fusiform cells crucial for facial recognition. Serotonin, which affects mood and social behavior, is notably involved in modulating the activities of these lobes.

Interactions among these lobes create a cohesive neural symphony that enables complex responses to stimuli. Neural pathways interlinking the lobes facilitate communication and coordination, ensuring that sensory input is quickly and efficiently processed into appropriate behavioral responses. For instance, when learning to play an instrument, the frontal lobe's decision-making works in conjunction with the temporal lobe's sound processing and the parietal lobe's spatial reasoning to coordinate hand movements.

Neural plasticity, the brain's ability to reorganize itself by forming new neural connections, plays a crucial role in each lobe. This adaptability is fundamental in learning new skills and recovering from injuries. For example, after a stroke affects parts of the frontal lobe, other areas of the brain can adapt to take over lost functions, highlighting the brain's remarkable ability to repair and modify itself.

Disruptions in the typical functioning of these lobes, such as from trauma or disease, can lead to profound neurological disorders. Alzheimer's disease, for instance, often begins in the temporal lobe, impairing memory before progressing to other areas. Understanding the specific functions and neurochemical environments of each lobe not only aids in diagnosing such conditions but also in developing targeted therapies that address the distinct pathologies involved.

In conclusion, the cerebral cortex's lobes represent a complex, interdependent network, central to our interaction with the world. Disruptions in their functions can lead to diverse psychological and neurological conditions, emphasizing the importance of this knowledge in medical science for diagnostic and therapeutic purposes.

Imagine watching a ballet dancer during rehearsal, where every motion is a testament to flawless timing, precise movements, and impeccable coordination. This scene perfectly mirrors the function of the cerebellum in the human brain. Just as the dancer executes each spin and step with practiced grace, the cerebellum manages our body's motor movements, ensuring that each physical action is smoothly carried out.

The cerebellum, much like the choreographer of a ballet, orchestrates movements that require a high degree of precision. It adjusts and refines motor signals, similar to how a dancer fine-tunes their performance to achieve elegance and fluidity. For instance, when a ballet dancer leaps, it's not just about the jump. The positioning of their arms, the timing of the take-off, and the softness of the landing are all meticulously coordinated. Similarly, the cerebellum coordinates how and when muscles activate during a run, or how our fingers move when typing on a keyboard.

Just as a ballet requires hours of practice for the steps to become second nature, our movements become smoother through the cerebellum's ability to learn and adapt physically. A dancer's rehearsal refines their performance over time, with muscle memory building to integrate steps into seamless sequences. In parallel, the cerebellum adjusts and perfects our movements, learning from repeated actions to enhance motor skills.

Ultimately, the cerebellum's role extends beyond mere movement, influencing our balance and spatial awareness, just as a dancer must be acutely aware of their space and posture. Understanding the cerebellum through the lens of ballet not only highlights its intricate functionality but also underscores its elegance, much like the poignant beauty of a perfectly executed pirouette. This analogy bridges the gap between a complex biological concept and an artful expression familiar to us all, helping to illuminate the intricate dance of our neurons in a way that resonates with our everyday experiences.

Here is the breakdown of the neural mechanisms within the cerebellum responsible for movement coordination:

- **Neural Circuits**: These circuits are fundamental to how the cerebellum controls and coordinates movement.
- **Mossy Fibers**: These fibers originate from various regions, including the spinal cord and the brainstem. They enter the cerebellum and synapse onto granule cells located within the granular layer. These fibers bring sensory and motor information to the cerebellum, serving as a primary input source.
- **Climbing Fibers**: Originating from the inferior olivary nucleus in the brainstem, these fibers form powerful, direct connections with Purkinje cells. Each climbing fiber wraps around a single Purkinje cell, influencing it through complex spikes, crucial for error teaching and motor learning.
- **Purkinje Cells**: These large neurons receive inputs from both mossy and climbing fibers. Purkinje cells integrate these signals and send inhibitory outputs to deep cerebellar nuclei. The output from these nuclei is critical in modulating activity in the motor cortex and brainstem, thus fine-tuning movement.

- **Signal Processing**:
    - The cerebellum processes signals in a precise loop essential for motor coordination:
        - Motor commands from the cerebral cortex are sent to the cerebellum via mossy fibers.
        - The cerebellum processes these commands, compares them with actual motor performance, and adjusts the commands to reduce errors.

- The refined commands are sent back to the motor cortex and spinal cord, enhancing the execution of movements.

- **Learning and Adaptation**:
- Synaptic plasticity within the cerebellar cortex plays a significant role in adapting and learning new motor tasks.
- Long-term depression (LTD) and long-term potentiation (LTP) at synapses, particularly those involving Purkinje cells, adjust the strength of synaptic connections based on feedback, improving movement accuracy over time.

- **Error Correction**:
- The cerebellum continually receives feedback on the discrepancies between intended movement and actual movement.
- This error feedback is processed mainly through the climbing fibers that adjust the output of the Purkinje cells.
- Such adjustments refine motor output, similar to how a dance instructor corrects a dancer's postures and movements, ensuring that performances are precise and well-coordinated.

This detailed list outlines the complex yet fascinating ways in which the cerebellum plays a pivotal role in our ability to execute coordinated and refined movements. Understanding these components provides insight into not just how we move, but how we learn and perfect our movements over time.

The brainstem, often regarded as the lifeline of the nervous system, plays a vital role in sustaining life-sustaining processes such as breathing and heart rate control. At its core, this part of the brain connects the cerebrum above to the spinal cord below, acting as a conduit through which all signals must pass.

Breathing, a function vital for life, is regulated by the medulla oblongata, a component of the brainstem. This area automatically controls the rate and depth of breathing by monitoring carbon dioxide levels in the blood and signaling the respiratory muscles accordingly. For instance, during intense exercise, carbon dioxide levels increase, and the medulla oblongata responds by accelerating breathing to maintain a balanced internal environment.

Similarly, the brainstem is crucial in managing heart rate. The medulla oblongata houses the cardiac control center, which fine-tunes the heart's pace to match the body's demands. When an individual experiences a fright, adrenaline released into the bloodstream signals this control center. In response, it quickens the heart rate, ensuring that muscles receive more oxygen-rich blood rapidly.

These critical functions underscore the brainstem's role as the nervous system's lifeline. By managing essential tasks like breathing and heart regulation, it upholds the body's capability to respond to varying conditions and maintain homeostasis.

In summary, the brainstem not only supports basic life

functions but also enables the body to dynamically adapt to changes, both internal and external. Understanding these operations illuminates the seamless integration of numerous processes that keep the human body functioning efficiently. This knowledge not only enhances one's appreciation of human physiology but also emphasizes the interconnectedness and precision of our nervous system's operations.

Let's take a deeper look at the sophisticated neural pathways within the medulla oblongata, focusing on their roles in heart rate and breathing control. This exploration provides a clearer understanding of how these critical functions are managed at a cellular level.

The medulla oblongata houses various specialized neurons that regulate autonomic functions. For breathing, neurons within the respiratory center of the medulla generate rhythmic patterns and adjust breathing rates based on the body's carbon dioxide levels. These neurons are sensitive to pH changes in the blood that result from shifts in carbon dioxide levels, adjusting the respiratory rate to maintain balance.

For heart rate control, the cardiac center comprises neurons that respond to the body's demands via signals from the nervous system and circulating hormones. These neurons monitor the body's condition and send signals to either speed up or slow down the heart rate. The neurotransmitters involved, mainly acetylcholine and noradrenaline, play pivotal roles. Acetylcholine slows the heart rate when the body is at rest, while noradrenaline increases the heart rate during stress or exercise.

Regarding receptors, the cardiac control center mainly interacts with muscarinic receptors in response to acetylcholine, and adrenergic receptors in response to noradrenaline. These receptors modulate the heart's activity efficiently, ensuring that it responds accurately to current body conditions.

Furthermore, the feedback loops between the medulla oblongata and both the heart and lungs are crucial for maintaining homeostasis. These loops allow for continuous monitoring and adjustments. For instance, if blood pressure falls, sensors in blood vessels send signals to the medulla, which then commands an increase in heart rate via adrenergic pathways, restoring blood pressure levels.

Understanding these intricate connections and mechanisms highlights the precision of our body's internal regulation systems and enhances our appreciation for the complex yet seamless operations that keep us alive and well. This foundational knowledge is key to approaching more advanced topics in human physiology and medical studies, ensuring a solid groundwork for further exploration into human health and disease.

Imagine the internet, a vast network where millions of bits of information speed across the globe in mere seconds, reaching their destinations through a complex web of connections. Just as web servers and routers play crucial roles in directing data through the right paths, so does the brain with its intricate network of neurons and synapses. In this sprawling neural network, messages are electrical impulses and chemical signals, traversing axons and dendrites to evoke responses from muscle movements to thought processes.

Each neuron in the brain can be compared to a mini-router, receiving, processing, and sending information packets in the form of neurotransmitters across synapses—the brain's version of network cables. This neurotransmission process ensures that messages are delivered efficiently, allowing for quick reflexes, immediate decision making, and complex emotional responses.

This analogy isn't just fascinating for its simplicity; it highlights the crucial role of connectivity in both networks. Just as a broken router or a severed internet cable can disrupt communication and data flow, disruptions in neural pathways can lead to physical and cognitive impairments. Understanding this parallel helps illuminate not just how the brain's communication system works, but also its vulnerability and the critical need for its protection and care.

Thus, when we discuss the brain's neural network, we're not just exploring biological facts; we're unraveling the foundation of every human action and thought, mirrored elegantly by the digital communications that underpin our modern world. This perspective not only aids in comprehending the brain's complex functionality but also connects it to the everyday digital experiences that shape our lives.

Here is the breakdown of the key neurotransmitters involved in neural communication, focusing on their roles, interactions, and the specific types of neurons they affect:

- **Glutamate**:
  - **Role**: Glutamate acts as the primary excitatory neurotransmitter in the brain, playing a critical role in amplifying the excitatory signals between neurons. It is crucial for synaptic plasticity, which underpins learning and memory.
  - **Sources**: Glutamate is released by numerous types of neurons throughout the brain, particularly those within the cerebral cortex and hippocampus, areas highly involved in cognitive processes.
  - **Receptors**:
    - **AMPA**: AMPA receptors swiftly respond to glutamate, leading to fast excitatory postsynaptic potentials that enhance communication between neurons.
    - **NMDA**: NMDA receptors play a crucial role in synaptic plasticity and memory function. These receptors are unique as they require both ligand binding and a pre-existing electrical gradient to activate.

- **GABA**:
  - **Role**: Gamma-aminobutyric acid (GABA) serves as the main inhibitory neurotransmitter in the brain, essential for balancing neuronal activity by reducing excessive excitability and thus preventing neurodegeneration.
  - **Sources**: GABA is primarily secreted by interneurons in the brain, which strategically modulate the activity of other neurons in various brain circuits.

- **Receptors**:
  - **GABA A**: These receptors respond quickly to GABA binding, allowing chloride ions to flow into the neuron, which typically results in inhibitory postsynaptic potentials that diminish neuronal activity.
  - **GABA B**: These metabotropic receptors are slower to respond and often lead to longer-lasting inhibitory effects through secondary messenger systems that further regulate neuronal activity.

- **Dopamine**:
  - **Role**: Dopamine is a versatile neurotransmitter known for its double duty in facilitating neural communication and modulating the reward centers of the brain, influencing both movement and emotional responses.
  - **Sources**: Dopamine is predominantly synthesized in the substantia nigra and ventral tegmental area, critical regions involved in reward, motivation, and fine motor control.
  - **Receptors**:
    - **D1**: These receptors are generally stimulatory, linked to the production of cyclic AMP, and are involved in modulating the brain's reward system.
    - **D2**: In contrast, D2 receptors can be inhibitory and are implicated in modulating the release of other neurotransmitters, thus playing a key role in behavior and cognition.

By detailing these neurotransmitters and their interactions, we illuminate the intricate pathways similar to data traveling across the internet. This exploration helps us appreciate the sophisticated biochemical dynamics that power every thought, decision, and action, enriching our understanding of the human brain's remarkable capabilities.

Exploring the anatomy of the brain reveals just how integral this organ is to every aspect of human life, controlling everything from basic motor functions to complex cognitive processes. The brain is comprised of various structures such as the cerebrum, cerebellum, and brainstem, each playing distinct and critical roles. The cerebrum, for instance, is responsible for higher cognitive functions such as reasoning, emotions, and learning, while the cerebellum regulates coordination and precision in our physical movements, and the brainstem governs essential involuntary processes like breathing and heart rate.

Understanding the brain's intricate structure and functionality not only deepens our comprehension of human biology but also highlights the remarkable capacity of the brain to adapt and evolve. This organ's complexity is evident in its ability to rewire itself — a phenomenon known as neuroplasticity — which allows it to recover from injuries and adjust to new learning experiences.

Reflecting on the importance of the brain, it is clear that this organ is not just an anatomical marvel but also a pivotal element of our identity and behavior. Knowledge of brain anatomy is crucial not only for medical and psychological fields but also enriches our understanding of what it means to be human, influencing everything from educational strategies to ethical considerations in both medicine and daily life. Thus, diving into the brain's anatomy is not merely an academic pursuit but a journey into the very essence of human capability and resilience.

NEUROCHEMISTRY AND NEUROTRANSMITTERS

Neurochemistry and neurotransmitters constitute the communication network of the brain, a complex system responsible for governing our thoughts, emotions, and actions. By exploring these biochemical messengers and the mechanisms by which they operate, we unlock crucial insights into human behavior and health. Neurotransmitters such as dopamine and serotonin influence everything from our mood to our ability to learn and remember. Misbalances in these chemicals are linked to various psychological conditions, illustrating the significant impact these substances have on our daily lives. This chapter aims to clarify these intricate processes in an accessible manner, ensuring that the concepts of neurochemistry are not just understood but appreciated in their full capacity. Understanding this can lead to better mental health management and provide a foundation for further exploration into how our brains shape our lives. With each section, we will dismantle complex scientific principles into clear, impactful knowledge, making this fascinating topic approachable and relevant to everyone curious about the inner workings of their own minds.

Neurotransmitters are the brain's chemical messengers, fundamental to transmitting signals within the nervous system. These substances are classified broadly into two categories: excitatory and inhibitory. Excitatory neurotransmitters, such as glutamate, promote the transmission of impulses, essentially telling neurons to activate. Inhibitory neurotransmitters, like GABA (gamma-aminobutyric acid), do the opposite—they prevent transmissions, keeping the neurons at rest.

Each neurotransmitter has a specific set of receptors with which it interacts, similar to a key fitting into a lock. This specificity ensures that messages are relayed accurately and efficiently within the brain, organizing a myriad of functions from simple muscle contractions to complex emotions. For instance, dopamine, a neurotransmitter linked with pleasure and motivation, has its receptors positioned in brain pathways where it plays a notable role in enhancing feelings of enjoyment and reinforcement, encouraging us to repeat behaviors that are rewarding.

Understanding these roles and classifications helps underline how crucial neurotransmitters are for daily brain function—they regulate not just how someone feels at any given moment but also influence long-term psychological and neurological functions. For example, serotonin impacts mood, sleep, and appetite, and imbalances in its levels are linked to depression and anxiety, thus illustrating the profound effect neurotransmitters have on overall health and well-being.

This information not only deepens one's understanding of how the brain operates but also emphasizes the necessity of maintaining a healthy neurotransmitter balance for optimal mental and physical health. By grasping these details, one can appreciate how the ongoing research and advancements in neurochemistry could lead to better management and treatment of various neurological disorders, revealing the significant implications of neurotransmitters in everyday life.

Let's take a deeper look at how neurotransmitters engage with their respective receptors within the brain's neurons and analyze the complexities of their interactions that greatly influence both brain function and behavior.

- **Receptor Binding**:
- **Glutamate**: When glutamate, the principal excitatory neurotransmitter, binds to its receptors (such as AMPA and NMDA receptors), it prompts these receptor channels to open. This opening allows positively charged ions like sodium (Na+) and calcium (Ca2+) to flow into the neuron, causing a depolarization of the neuron's membrane.
- **GABA**: In contrast, GABA, the main inhibitory neurotransmitter, typically binds to GABA_A receptors. This binding event allows the influx of negatively charged chloride ions (Cl-) into the neuron, leading to hyperpolarization. This hyperpolarization makes the neuron less likely to fire an action potential (nerve impulse).

- **Signal Transduction Mechanisms**:
- Binding of neurotransmitters to their receptors typically triggers a cascade of biochemical reactions inside the neuron. For glutamate receptors, the flow of Ca2+ can activate various intracellular signaling pathways, often involving secondary messengers like cyclic AMP (cAMP), which further influence cell functions and gene expression.
- For GABA, the increased chloride influx usually results in an increase in negative charge inside the neuron, further stabilizing the membrane potential and inhibiting cellular

excitability.

- **Neuronal Response**:
    - The changes incited by these neurotransmitters at the receptor level immediately affect the neuron's electrical status. In the case of excitatory signals (like those from glutamate), the neuron's membrane potential may reach a threshold that triggers action potentials, facilitating the rapid propagation of signals along the neuron and onto other connected neurons.
    - Inhibitory signals (like those from GABA), however, increase the neuron's membrane potential's negativity, inhibiting action potentials and thus reducing signal propagation, which is crucial in controlling overexcitation in neural circuits.

- **Feedback Loops and Modulation**:
    - Neurons have mechanisms to regulate the sensitivity and density of neurotransmitter receptors based on the neuron's activity level. This modulation helps maintain homeostasis and adaptively modulate neuron responsivity depending on stimulus demand.
    - Additionally, feedback loops involving the neurotransmitter release can either enhance or inhibit further neurotransmitter release. For example, an excess of a neurotransmitter might trigger feedback mechanisms that inhibit further release or decrease receptor sensitivity, to prevent overstimulation and potential neuronal damage.

By understanding these receptor-neurotransmitter interactions and their consequent effects on neuronal activity and communications, we gain profound insights into the neuronal basis for a multitude of brain functions and behaviors. This exploration not only emphasizes the complexity and finesse of our nervous system but also anchors our understanding of neurophysiological processes comprehensively and pragmatically.

Imagine you're in a bustling classroom where students are silently passing notes to each other. Each note contains a message that needs to reach a specific classmate. This scene is surprisingly similar to how neurons in the brain communicate through synaptic transmission.

In this analogy, each student represents a neuron. The note is similar to a neurotransmitter, a chemical messenger crucial for carrying information. When a student (neuron) decides to send a message, they write a note (synthesize a neurotransmitter) and pass it across the room via a series of handoffs (this represents the synaptic cleft, the small space between neurons). The student receiving the note takes it, reads it (just like a receptor receiving and responding to a neurotransmitter), and decides how to respond, perhaps by writing another note or by performing some action based on the message received.

Just as the note's content affects the recipient's response—whether they smile, frown, or write a reply—the type of neurotransmitter released influences how the receiving neuron will react. Some neurotransmitters might excite the receiving neuron, prompting it to pass along the message (like an intriguing rumor that spreads quickly through the classroom). Other neurotransmitters might inhibit the neuron, making it less likely to 'speak up' or continue the chain (similar to a directive to stop passing notes).

This simple classroom activity underscores not only the process of sending and receiving messages but also the importance of correct message delivery. Miscommunications in this system—similar to someone intercepting a note and changing its contents—can lead to errors, just as dysfunctions in synaptic transmission can lead to neurological disorders or diseases.

Through this familiar scenario, we gain a clearer picture of the elegant, yet highly complex, interactions that drive communication within the brain, shaping our thoughts, actions, and reactions in countless ways.

Here is the breakdown of the key neurotransmitters and their interactions with specific receptors, along with the subsequent cellular responses that drive synaptic transmission in the brain:

- **Types of Neurotransmitters**:
    - **Glutamate**: This neurotransmitter predominantly acts as an excitatory signal in the brain, enhancing the likelihood that the receiving neuron will fire an action potential. It is vital for processes such as learning and memory.
    - **GABA (Gamma-Aminobutyric Acid)**: In contrast to glutamate, GABA serves primarily as an inhibitory neurotransmitter. By binding to its receptors, it decreases the probability that the post-synaptic neuron will fire, thus

calming neural activity.
- **Dopamine**: Known for its role in the reward system of the brain, dopamine modulation affects various brain functions, notably influencing behaviors linked to pleasure, motivation, and fine motor control.
- **Serotonin**: This neurotransmitter plays a crucial role in regulating mood, appetite, and sleep cycles. Its imbalance is often linked with depression and anxiety disorders.

- **Receptor Interaction**:
- **Ionotropic Receptors**: These receptors directly control the opening of ion channels on the post-synaptic neuron's membrane, leading to quick changes in the neuron's membrane potential. For example, glutamate often binds to these receptors to excite neurons rapidly.
- **Metabotropic Receptors**: These receptors operate indirectly, initiating a series of intracellular reactions that involve second messengers such as cAMP (cyclic Adenosine Monophosphate). These reactions eventually influence neuronal activity by modulating various cellular processes over a longer duration.

- **Cellular Response**:
- When neurotransmitters bind to ionotropic receptors, the immediate response is either an influx or efflux of ions like Na^+ or Cl^-, which alters the electrical charge across the neuronal membrane. This change can either trigger an action potential if the neurotransmitter is excitatory (like glutamate) or prevent one if inhibitory (like GABA).
- Interaction with metabotropic receptors doesn't directly change the membrane potential but instead affects the neuron through more complex biochemical pathways

that can change the neuron's excitability or function over a longer term, affecting everything from gene expression to cellular metabolism.

By understanding these detailed interactions and responses, readers gain a clearer insight into how neurons communicate among themselves through a sophisticated chemical language. This detailed exploration not only enriches the comprehension of basic brain functions but also illustrates the biochemical basis for many psychological and neurological phenomena, from simple reflexes to complex emotions and behaviors.

Neurotransmitter imbalances in the brain can lead directly to various psychological conditions, influencing both mood and behavior profoundly. To understand this connection, consider neurotransmitters as the brain's chemical messengers; they transmit signals across the brain that help regulate not only our feelings and mood but also our decisions and physical responses. When these chemical messengers are out of balance, the brain's usual functioning can be disrupted.

For example, serotonin, often labeled the 'feel-good' neurotransmitter, plays a crucial role in stabilizing our mood, feelings of well-being, and happiness. Low levels of serotonin are commonly associated with depression. Similarly, dopamine, another significant neurotransmitter, affects our sensation of pleasure and reward and is linked with motivation. Dysregulated dopamine levels are observed in individuals with addiction and schizophrenia, indicating too much or too little dopamine can profoundly affect cognition and behavior.

Moreover, consider norepinephrine, which regulates stress and anxiety. An imbalance in this neurotransmitter can lead to anxiety disorders, characterized by excessive fear, worry, and nervousness. Understanding these links underlines the critical impact that balanced neurotransmitter levels have on maintaining mental health and functional behavior.

This explanation illuminates how neurotransmitter imbalances can disrupt normal life, leading to psychological conditions that might affect one's ability to function effectively in daily activities. By grasping the science behind neurotransmitter functions and their impacts, we can better comprehend how treatments like medications or lifestyle changes aimed at restoring this balance might improve mental health outcomes. Thus, these biochemical insights not only heighten our understanding but also empower us with knowledge to manage and potentially mitigate these conditions effectively.

Neurotransmitters are synthesized in various parts of the brain, depending on their type. For instance, serotonin is predominantly produced in the raphe nuclei located within the brainstem. The synthesis involves enzymes such as tryptophan hydroxylase, which converts the amino acid tryptophan into 5-hydroxytryptophan, later transformed into serotonin. Factors influencing the rate of production include genetic variations, diet, and overall health, including stress levels which can disrupt normal production processes.

Receptors play a critical role in how neurotransmitters affect neuron function. Neurotransmitters bind to specific receptors on the surface of neurons – ionotropic receptors quickly change the neuron's membrane potential and initiate an immediate response by opening ion channels, while metabotropic receptors affect the neuron through slower, more complex pathways involving second messengers. An imbalance in neurotransmitter levels can lead to inappropriate activation or inhibition of these receptors, disrupting normal neural communication and contributing to symptoms of mental health disorders.

At the cellular level, these disruptions can alter the firing patterns of neurons, leading to a domino effect across neural networks that regulate mood, thought processes, and emotional responses. For instance, a deficiency in serotonin can lead to decreased neuron activity in pathways that regulate mood, potentially resulting in depression. Similarly, excess dopamine in certain brain pathways is associated with symptoms of schizophrenia, such as hallucinations and delusions.

Addressing these imbalances, treatments involve strategies aimed at restoring normal neurotransmitter levels and receptor function. Pharmacotherapy may include medications like selective serotonin reuptake inhibitors (SSRIs) that increase serotonin levels in the brain by blocking its reabsorption in the synapses. Psychotherapy can provide strategies to manage stress, which can help normalize neurotransmitter function. Additionally, lifestyle changes such as regular exercise and a balanced diet can support neurotransmitter production and balance.

Understanding these biochemical mechanisms is vital to comprehending how subtle changes in the molecular level can significantly impact overall psychological health and behavior. This knowledge not only enhances our grasp of mental health disorders but also underscores the importance of targeted treatment approaches to manage and potentially reverse the adverse effects of neurotransmitter imbalances.

Just like a well-oiled machine operates at peak efficiency, our brain functions best when its neurotransmitters are well-balanced. This balance can be significantly enhanced through thoughtful dietary choices and regular exercise, much like regular maintenance ensures smooth running of a machine.

For starters, incorporating foods rich in essential nutrients can bolster neurotransmitter production. Omega-3 fatty acids, found abundantly in fish like salmon, are known to support brain function and mood regulation. Similarly, foods rich in tryptophan – such as turkey and eggs – provide the building blocks for serotonin, a key neurotransmitter that influences our mood and emotional well-being.

On the exercise front, engaging in regular physical activity acts like greasing the cogs of our brain's machinery. Exercise increases blood flow to the brain, which helps to nourish neurons with oxygen and nutrients while also encouraging the release of various neurotransmitters including endorphins, often dubbed the 'feel-good' chemicals. This not only uplifts mood but also sharpens cognition and reduces stress, which can disrupt neurotransmitter balance.

Together, a balanced diet and regular physical activity ensure that our brain's neurotransmitters are produced, released, and function as needed, similar to keeping a machine in its best possible condition. By taking care of our diet and ensuring regular exercise, we can effectively tune our brain's intricate system for optimal performance, making the process of managing and improving mental health not just necessary, but also enjoyable.

Let's take a deeper look at how specific nutrients and physical activities influence neurotransmitter levels and synaptic functions, offering actionable ways to positively impact brain health.

- **Omega-3 Fatty Acids**:
Omega-3 fatty acids, particularly EPA and DHA, play a crucial role in maintaining the fluidity of cell membranes, which is essential for the optimal functioning of neuron receptors and other enzymatic proteins involved in neurotransmitter synthesis and release. These fatty acids are incorporated into the phospholipid bilayer of neuron cell membranes, enhancing their flexibility and permeability. This improvement in membrane properties facilitates more efficient neurotransmitter binding and release, and better signal transduction across synapses. Furthermore, omega-3s have anti-inflammatory properties that reduce neural inflammation, a condition often linked with depressed mood and cognitive decline.

- **Tryptophan to Serotonin Conversion**:
Serotonin synthesis starts with the amino acid tryptophan, which crosses the blood-brain barrier with the help of a transport protein. Once inside the brain, tryptophan undergoes a series of enzymatic reactions. The first key enzyme, tryptophan hydroxylase, converts tryptophan into 5-hydroxytryptophan (5-HTP), which is then decarboxylated by the enzyme aromatic L-amino acid decarboxylase to produce serotonin. This process is nutrient-dependent; for instance, vitamin B6 is a cofactor for the decarboxylation step. Hence, dietary intake of both tryptophan-rich foods, like turkey and eggs, and B-vitamins can significantly influence serotonin levels, impacting mood and emotional well-being.

- **Physical Exercise and Neurotransmitter Release**:
Engaging in physical exercise stimulates the release of various neurotransmitters, including endorphins—the body's natural painkillers and mood elevators—and serotonin, which enhances feelings of well-being and happiness. Exercise increases blood flow to the brain, which improves oxygen and nutrient supply to neurons, supporting their health and function. It also activates the sympathetic nervous system, triggering the release of certain neurotransmitters and enhancing their synthesis. Regular physical activity increases the expression of trophic factors like BDNF (Brain-Derived Neurotrophic Factor), which promotes the survival and growth of neurons, further benefiting neurotransmitter systems and overall brain health.

By understanding these mechanisms, we can see how diet

and exercise are not just about physical health but are crucial for maintaining neurotransmitter balance and enhancing brain function. This approach to daily habits can be likened to performing regular maintenance on a machine; just as consistent care keeps a machine running smoothly, a balanced diet and regular exercise keep our brain's neurotransmitter systems functioning optimally, improving our mental health and cognitive abilities.

This chapter has unveiled the intricate world of neurochemistry and neurotransmitters, illustrating how these microscopic agents orchestrate vast networks of neural communication. By appreciating the fundamental roles that neurotransmitters play—from facilitating synaptic transmissions to shaping our emotions and behaviors—we equip ourselves with a deeper understanding of human biology. The insights gained here spotlight the crucial balance of chemical messengers, which, when disrupted, can lead to a spectrum of psychological and neurological conditions.

A comprehension of neurochemistry extends beyond academic curiosity; it has tangible implications for personal health. Recognizing how dietary choices, exercise, and other lifestyle factors can influence neurotransmitter activity empowers us to make informed decisions that enhance our mental and physical well-being. Moreover, understanding these biochemical underpinnings enhances our ability to empathize with and support those affected by mental health challenges, bridging the gap between scientific knowledge and compassionate care.

Ultimately, the study of neurochemistry and neurotransmitters invites us to marvel at the complexity and adaptability of the human brain, encouraging a continuous pursuit of knowledge that enriches both scientific and personal realms. This convergence of science and everyday life not only informs but also inspires, driving forward our collective quest for enlightenment and improved well-being.

COGNITIVE FUNCTIONS

The human brain, a marvel of nature, is equipped with powerful cognitive functions that guide memory, learning, decision-making, and problem-solving. These functions are not just academic topics; they are core tools that help us navigate daily challenges, enhance our interactions, and shape our future. Understanding the mechanics of these capabilities reveals how we can apply them more effectively and improve our mental agility to overcome obstacles, large and small. This chapter unravels the complexities of the brain's cognitive processes in an accessible format, illustrating how deeply intertwined these functions are with every aspect of our lives. By exploring how these processes work, we not only gain insight into our brain's impressive abilities but also develop strategies to harness these powers, enhancing our decision-making and problem-solving skills in personal and professional contexts.

Memory in the human brain functions through three key stages: encoding, storage, and retrieval. Encoding begins when we first encounter information. For example, when learning a new phone number, the brain initially processes the sequence of numbers during this phase. This is similar to typing data into a computer—input that needs to be saved for later use.

Once encoded, the information moves to the storage phase. Think of this stage as saving the typed data on a computer's hard drive. The brain categorizes this information into short-term or long-term memory, much like data saved on different forms of digital storage. Short-term memory is like a computer's RAM, temporarily holding information for quick access and use. In contrast, long-term memory compares to a hard drive, where information can be stored indefinitely.

Finally, retrieval occurs when the brain accesses this stored information. Returning to the phone number example, recalling the number when needed mirrors pulling a file from a computer's hard drive back onto the screen to be viewed or used.

Understanding these stages helps to appreciate how the brain manages information, much like a sophisticated, organic computer. This insight not only enhances comprehension of one's memory capabilities but also opens paths to refining memory retention strategies, such as repetition to strengthen storage or creating associations to aid retrieval. By dissecting these mechanisms, the complexities of memory become tangible aspects of everyday life, empowering individuals with the knowledge to harness and optimize their cognitive processes.

Let's take a deeper look at the biochemistry of memory stages in the human brain, dissecting the roles of specific neurotransmitters and the impact of certain external influences on memory processing.

- **Biochemistry of Encoding**:
At the encoding phase, neurotransmitters play a pivotal

role in how memories are initially formed. Acetylcholine, for example, is crucial for attention and plays a significant role in enhancing the strength of the signals between neurons, particularly in the hippocampus, the area of the brain vital for forming new memories. Additionally, dopamine is released during pleasurable situations and enhances the encoding of memory by increasing synaptic plasticity. This process strengthens the connections between neurons, making it easier to recall this information later.

- **Storage Mechanisms**:

When a memory moves from short-term to long-term storage, several structural changes occur at the synapse level. This is primarily facilitated by a process known as long-term potentiation (LTP). LTP involves the strengthening of the synaptic connections between neurons, with the protein CREB (cAMP response element-binding protein) playing a critical role. CREB helps in the transcription of new proteins that solidify the memory within the neural network, transforming a short-term memory into a long-term one.

- **Retrieval Dynamics**:

Retrieval involves re-accessing the information stored within the brain. This process heavily relies on the prefrontal cortex, which helps in organizing and retrieving memories. Stress, however, can affect this process significantly. Cortisol, a stress hormone, can impair the retrieval process by destabilizing the neural networks involved in memory recall, making it more challenging to access certain memories.

Understanding these intricate mechanisms offers us not just a window into the profound complexities of our cognitive functions but also underscores the critical influences of our daily experiences and emotional states on our memory systems. By engaging with this knowledge, one gains a greater appreciation and control over the factors that affect our memory, ultimately empowering us to optimize our cognitive health and performance.

Imagine you're at the gym, lifting weights to build and strengthen your muscles. Each time you exercise, your muscles undergo small changes; fibers tear slightly and rebuild stronger. This process is quite similar to how synaptic plasticity works in our brains during learning.

Just as lifting weights strengthens muscles, engaging in mental exercises and learning activities strengthens the connections between neurons in the brain. These connections, or synapses, are like the muscle fibers; they grow stronger and more efficient with use. When you learn something new, your brain fires a specific pattern of neurons. The repeated activation of these neurons during learning enhances their ability to transmit signals to each other, a phenomenon known as synaptic plasticity.

Also, just as consistent workouts increase muscle size and power, repeated neural activity through learning solidifies these connections, making the transmission of information faster and more efficient. This biological process underlies learning and memory, enabling not just the storage of information but also the enhancement of cognitive abilities overall.

Understanding synaptic plasticity through this analogy highlights why regular 'mental workouts' are just as crucial as physical ones. They are essential for maintaining a healthy, responsive, and adaptable brain, ensuring that just like well-conditioned muscles, our cognitive functions can handle challenges more effectively as they arise. This also showcases the beauty and ongoing capability of our brain to adapt and grow, much like our muscles do, in response to new information and experiences.

Here is the breakdown of the synaptic plasticity process, which details the biochemical changes at the synaptic level during learning:

- **Neurotransmitter Role**:
    - **Glutamate**: Often acts as the primary excitatory neurotransmitter in synaptic plasticity. It binds to NMDA and AMPA receptors, facilitating calcium influx and strengthening the synaptic connections.
    - **GABA**: Functions as the main inhibitory neurotransmitter, balancing the excitatory signals by reducing neuronal activity, which is essential in sculpting neural circuits during learning.

- **Synaptic Changes**:
    - **Density of Postsynaptic Receptors**: Learning and repeated stimulus exposure often lead to an increase in the number and density of postsynaptic receptors, enhancing synaptic efficacy.
    - **Dendritic Spines**: Structural modifications occur in dendritic spines (protrusions on dendrites where synapses

are located), which can change in size and shape, thereby affecting their connectivity and strength.

- **Signal Enhancements**:
  - **Receptor Sensitivity**: Changes in the properties of synaptic receptors can alter their sensitivity to neurotransmitters, improving the synapse's responsiveness to neurotransmitter signals.
  - **Synaptic Connections**: New synaptic connections may form, and existing connections may be strengthened or weakened, a process crucial for network reorganization and memory consolidation.

- **Long-Term Effects**:
  - **Long-Term Potentiation (LTP)**: This refers to the long-lasting improvement of signals between two neurons, resulting from synchronous stimulation. LTP is a primary mechanism behind the strengthening of memory.
  - **Long-Term Depression (LTD)**: In contrast to LTP, LTD involves a long-lasting decrease in synaptic strength, which is important for memory extinction and synaptic pruning.

By understanding these components, one can appreciate how learning involves not just the accumulation of knowledge but also significant structural and functional changes within the brain. This dynamic alteration enhances our cognitive capabilities and shapes how we interact with and perceive the world, making learning a continuous, life-shaping phenomenon.

The brain's decision-making process is remarkably similar to how a computer algorithm operates to produce the optimum outcome from a set of data. Initially, the brain gathers information, much like data inputs in a computer. This initial gathering involves sensory input and recalling relevant memories that provide context and comparison for decision-making.

Subsequently, the prefrontal cortex of the brain functions similarly to a processor in a computer, undertaking the role of analyzing this information. It evaluates potential outcomes and weighs the risks and benefits of each option. This is analogous to an algorithm in a computer running through possible solutions to select the most effective one based on predefined criteria.

Neurotransmitters play a crucial role in this phase—they act as messengers conveying signals across various parts of the brain, enhancing the communication necessary for solid decision-making. This can be thought of as the bandwidth in computer terms, which facilitates faster and more efficient data transfer, enabling quicker processing speeds.

Once the analysis is complete, the brain, like a computer, arrives at a decision by selecting the option that maximizes benefit while minimizing risks and other costs. The result is a decision that, ideally, represents the best possible choice given the available information—mirroring how sophisticated software might output the most effective solution to a problem based on the data it has analyzed.

Understanding this intricate process provides a deeper appreciation for the complexity and capability of both the human brain and advanced computing systems. It illuminates how our everyday decisions, seemingly simple on the surface, are backed by a profoundly complex cognitive mechanism—a process that is continuously refined through experiences and learning, much like how an algorithm can be trained and improved over time.

The decision-making process in the human brain is an intricate, multi-step operation, analogous to how a sophisticated computer algorithm processes data to reach conclusions. Here's a detailed breakdown of each component involved in this cognitive process:

- **Sensory Input**: Sensory information is the primary data input for the brain. Just as sensors in devices detect environmental stimuli, sensory organs—eyes, ears, skin, nose, and tongue—gather inputs from the surroundings. This information is then converted into neural signals that are sent to the brain, initiating the decision-making process. These signals are filtered through the thalamus, which prioritizes them before they reach the higher brain regions for further processing, much like a preliminary sorting of data in a computational model.

- **Neurotransmitter Functioning**: Neurotransmitters are biochemical substances that play a crucial role in transmitting signals across neurons at synapses. Dopamine and serotonin are two key neurotransmitters that influence decision-making. Dopamine is often associated with reward and pleasure pathways; it enhances signal transmission that predicts positive outcomes, thereby encouraging decision-making aligned with those expected results. On the other hand, serotonin modulates mood, anxiety, and overall well-being, thereby inhibiting or dampening neural circuits in decision-making during high-stress or unfavorable conditions. This modulation by neurotransmitters parallels how bandwidth and data flow are managed in computational systems, ensuring that the processing speed and quality are maintained without overload.

- **Cortical Analysis**: The prefrontal cortex (PFC) acts similarly to a computer's central processing unit (CPU). It receives the filtered sensory data and the modulated signals influenced by neurotransmitters. In this cortical 'analysis phase,' the PFC evaluates potential outcomes, risks, and benefits associated with each possible decision. This evaluation involves complex neural circuits that compare current data with past experiences and potential future consequences. Executive functions housed in the PFC are crucial here; they help in focusing attention, overriding impulsive responses, and making calculated decisions based on logical reasoning and emotional assessment.

These components collectively ensure that decision-making is a balanced, informed process, integrating both emotional and rational data to come to a conclusion. By comparing this process to a computer algorithm, one can appreciate the precision and efficiency with which the human brain operates, as well as the complexity of the underlying neural mechanisms that enable everyday decisions, from the mundane to the critical. Understanding this helps highlight both the remarkable capabilities and the limitations of our cognitive processes, encouraging strategies to enhance decision-making skills.

Tackling a problem can often feel like piecing together a complex jigsaw puzzle. Initially, when you spread out all the pieces on a table, the task appears daunting, fragments scattered with little indication of the final image. This is much like facing a new challenge—everything seems disconnected at first glance. The process begins by identifying corner and edge pieces, establishing the framework, similar to grasping the overall scope and structure of a problem.

As you fit these initial pieces together, you start to work on specific sections, which can be likened to breaking down a larger problem into smaller, more manageable parts. This approach allows for focused thinking on one segment at a time, making the task less overwhelming. You might find a patch of blue sky in one corner or the green of a leaf in another. In problem-solving, these are the moments of insight or partial solutions that begin to form a coherent picture.

Gradually, as more pieces fit together, the image on the box—the big picture—begins to make sense in relation to the pieces you've been assembling. This reflects the importance of keeping the overall goal in mind while managing the details, ensuring that each step or solution aligns with the larger objective. Just as in a jigsaw puzzle, misplaced pieces can mislead or delay completion, incorrect or irrelevant solutions can divert resources and focus in real-world problem-solving.

Ultimately, the satisfaction of completing a jigsaw puzzle – snapping in the final piece and stepping back to admire the completed picture – mirrors the fulfillment of effectively solving a complex problem. Both processes require patience, a methodical approach, and an ability to see both the broad scope and intricate details. Understanding this analogy helps us appreciate the strategic and tactical aspects of problem-solving, empowering us to apply these skills across various challenges in our personal and professional lives.

Here is the breakdown on the cognitive processes involved in problem-solving, emphasizing how psychological aspects influence decision-making:

- **Initial Assessment**:
- Individuals first assess the complexity and familiarity of a problem. This initial overview helps in determining the approach and resources needed.
   - **Cognitive Biases**: During this phase, cognitive biases can significantly influence how the problem is perceived. Confirmation bias might lead someone to focus only on information that confirms their existing beliefs, whereas anchoring might result in over-reliance on the first piece of information encountered.

- **Strategy Development**:
- This phase involves formulating strategies to address the problem, utilizing logical reasoning and creative thinking.
   - **Pattern Recognition**: Part of strategy development includes recognizing patterns from past experiences which can inform the current approach.

- **Heuristic Methods**: Simplified processes that aid decision-making, such as breaking the problem down into smaller parts or using a trial-and-error method.
- **Experience and Knowledge**: Previous experiences and accumulated knowledge play a crucial role in shaping the strategies devised. These elements help in predicting potential pitfalls and in leveraging effective methods known to yield results.

- **Implementation and Evaluation**:
  - After strategizing, the proposed solutions are implemented to solve the problem.
  - **Feedback Loop**: Critical to this stage is the use of feedback, which helps in assessing the efficacy of the implemented solution. Feedback allows for real-time adjustments and improvements, ensuring that the approach remains aligned with solving the problem efficiently.

- **Continuous Improvement**:
  - Problem-solving is an iterative process. Each experience contributes to a deeper understanding and development of more refined strategies for future problems.
  - **Adapting Strategies Based on Outcomes**: Learning from what worked or did not work helps in refining problem-solving tactics. This adaptation can be crucial for dealing with more complex or similar future issues effectively.

This expanded content aims to provide a thorough understanding of the cognitive processes involved in problem-solving, highlighting the role of psychological factors in effective decision-making. By mastering these components, individuals are better equipped to tackle challenges methodically and successfully, whether in personal scenarios or within professional environments.

Enhancing cognitive functions is a vital aspect of maintaining mental agility and overall brain health. One effective way to boost these functions is through targeted exercises that stimulate different parts of the brain. For instance, engaging in puzzles like crosswords or Sudoku challenges problem-solving skills and enhances pattern recognition abilities. These activities foster neural connectivity, improving memory and the ability to process complex information swiftly.

Mindful practices, such as meditation, also play a crucial role in cognitive enhancement. Regular meditation helps in managing stress, which is known to impair cognitive functions. Moreover, it promotes better focus and concentration. For example, daily sessions of focused breathing or mindfulness can help an individual maintain mental clarity throughout the day, making tasks such as planning, decision-making, and multitasking more manageable and more precise.

Brain games, tailored to improve specific cognitive skills, offer another practical approach. These games often target memory, attention, and processing speed. For instance, memory matching games or apps designed to improve attention can lead to noticeable improvements in these areas. It's important to choose games that progressively increase in difficulty to ensure continuous cognitive challenge and growth.

Incorporating these activities into daily routines can be simple and enjoyable. Dedicate a few minutes to a puzzle during a coffee break or practice meditation during a quiet morning moment. Consistency is key, as the benefits of these cognitive exercises accrue over time, enhancing the brain's capacity to handle various cognitive tasks efficiently and effectively.

By understanding and applying these techniques, individuals not only bolster their cognitive capacities but also equip themselves with tools to improve their quality of life. These straightforward practices provide a foundational approach to nurturing and maintaining a sharp, responsive mind as part of a balanced, healthy lifestyle.

Throughout this chapter, we explored the critical role that cognitive functions play in our day-to-day lives and delved into techniques that enhance these functions. From engaging in brain-stimulating puzzles and games to integrating mindful practices into our routines, we've uncovered a variety of strategies designed to boost mental agility and overall brain health. Each method offers a distinct benefit, whether it's improving memory through targeted exercises or enhancing concentration and stress management through meditation.

As we move forward, it's essential to continue applying these cognitive strategies regularly. Just as with any skill, consistency is key to reaping the full benefits of cognitive exercises. Incorporating these practices into your daily life can lead to significant improvements in how you process information, solve problems, and make decisions.

I encourage you to keep exploring these cognitive enhancement techniques. Further learning and consistent practice can help you not only maintain but also advance your cognitive capabilities. By staying curious and proactive about your mental health, you ensure that your cognitive functions remain sharp and effective, empowering you to handle complex challenges with ease and confidence.

This journey into understanding and enhancing our cognitive abilities is ongoing. As new research emerges and our understanding of the brain deepens, so too will the strategies to optimize its function. Stay engaged, keep experimenting with new methods, and enjoy the process of sharpening your mind as you would any other vital skill.

EMOTIONS AND THE BRAIN

Emotions, those complex reactions that color our experiences and shape our interactions, are deeply rooted in the intricate workings of our brain. This chapter unravels the neurological tapestry that orchestrates our emotional lives by examining how certain brain regions contribute to the generation and regulation of emotions. Understanding this link between brain structure and emotional processes is not merely an academic pursuit. It holds practical significance in everyday life, informing how we manage stress, relate to others, and make decisions that align with our feelings.

By diving into the roles of key brain areas—the amygdala, the hippocampus, and the prefrontal cortex—we will explore the biological paths that lead to emotional responses. Such knowledge fosters a deeper appreciation of both the universality and the individuality of human emotions. It empowers us to more effectively interpret our own emotional experiences and those of others, enabling better communication, enhancing emotional intelligence, and promoting mental well-being.

Moving through these insights, the aim is to present clear, concise explanations that break down complex physiological mechanisms into fundamental concepts readily accessible to all. Whether you are a student, a professional, or simply curious about the workings of your own mind, this exploration into the emotional brain offers valuable perspectives that connect scientific knowledge with the fabric of everyday life.

The emotional landscape of the human brain is primarily sculpted by three pivotal structures: the amygdala, the hippocampus, and the prefrontal cortex, each playing distinct yet interconnected roles. The amygdala, often likened to a central alarm system, swiftly identifies emotional content in the stimuli we encounter, such as recognizing a threat. This rapid detection triggers an immediate emotional response, preparing the body for action—be it fight or flight.

Adjacent to this alarm system lies the hippocampus, pivotal not just for storing memories but for infusing them with emotional hues. It enables individuals to recall not only past events but also the associated feelings, enhancing the learning process from these experiences. For instance, recalling the warmth of a friendly gathering can encourage more social interactions.

At the helm of regulating these emotional responses is the prefrontal cortex, acting as an executive leader. This region moderates the impulses generated by the amygdala, applying rational thinking and situational context to fine-tune how one expresses and handles emotions. It decides if the initial fear triggered by the amygdala should be escalated or calmed based on logical assessment and past experiences stored in the hippocampus.

Together, these structures orchestrate a complex network of neural pathways that allow for nuanced emotional experiences and sophisticated behavioral outputs. By understanding how these parts of the brain interact to produce and regulate emotions, one gains profound insights into managing their emotional responses more effectively, leading to improved decision-making and interpersonal relations. This knowledge not only helps in appreciating the biological bases of emotions but also equips one with the understanding necessary to foster mental resilience and enhance emotional intelligence in daily life.

Let's take a deeper look at the intricate neural circuits and neurotransmitters that form the substrates for emotional processing between the amygdala, hippocampus, and prefrontal cortex. This detailed examination sheds light on their roles in shaping our emotional experiences.

Neural Pathways Connecting Key Brain Regions:
The amygdala, hippocampus, and prefrontal cortex are interconnected through complex neural pathways. Information about emotional stimuli first reaches the amygdala, which assesses emotional salience and quickly generates an initial emotional reaction. This reaction can include activation of the sympathetic nervous system—preparing for 'fight or flight.' The amygdala then communicates with the hippocampus to contextualize the emotional reaction based on past experiences and stored emotional memories.

Simultaneously, the amygdala sends signals to the prefrontal cortex, which is responsible for moderating these responses. The prefrontal cortex, using inputs from both the amygdala and hippocampus, evaluates the appropriateness of the emotional responses considering the current context and potential future outcomes. This area can enhance or suppress the initial emotional reactions initiated by the amygdala, leading to a more measured response.

Role of Neurotransmitters:
Neurotransmitters like serotonin and dopamine play pivotal roles within these pathways. Serotonin, often associated with mood regulation, modulates the intensity of neural signals passing between these regions, affecting the overall emotional tone. Higher levels of serotonin are linked with feelings of well-being and stability, whereas lower levels are often found in states of depression and anxiety.

Dopamine is critical in the 'reward' circuits of the brain, influencing aspects of reward-seeking behavior and pleasure. Dopamine levels can affect responses to positive stimuli and are integral in regulating emotions like joy and excitement.

Types of Emotional Responses and Physiological Processes:
The emotional responses modulated by these circuits cover a wide spectrum, such as fear, joy, and sadness. In reactions to fear, for instance, the amygdala activates faster and more instinctual responses, while the prefrontal cortex works to assess if the fear is rational and how to manage it effectively, damping down excessive responses if deemed unnecessary.

In moments of joy or happiness, dopamine release can enhance these pathways, leading to reinforcement of behaviors that provide pleasure or satisfaction. Conversely, sadness might be regulated differently, involving less dopamine transmission, which might influence motivational states.

Understanding these dynamics provides a clearer picture of how emotions are not just fleeting changes in mental states but are deeply rooted in our brain's architecture. This knowledge does not just enrich our insight into emotional processing; it also lays the groundwork for better mental health management, allowing us to understand fundamentally how our brains shape our emotional lives.

Imagine your brain has its own high-tech security system, with the amygdala acting as the vigilant security guard. This tiny, almond-shaped structure in your brain functions like the latest and fastest security alarm, expertly designed to detect any emotional stimuli or potential threats. When you encounter something unexpected — say, a sudden loud noise or an unnerving shadow in a dimly lit alley — it's the amygdala that instantly decides if these signals pose a threat, setting off alarms in your body before you're even fully aware of the danger.

This process is similar to a sophisticated security system that, upon detecting an intruder, sends out a rapid response to protect the home. The amygdala, in response to potential danger, triggers a cascade of biological reactions designed to ensure survival. This includes accelerating your heart rate, increasing blood flow to muscles, and heightening your senses—all part of the body's fight-or-flight response.

The critical role of the amygdala in our survival instincts is evident in how it prioritizes speed over detail. It quickly mobilizes a response with the basic information at hand, similar to how a security system might set off an alarm based on motion sensors without waiting to identify the intruder. This rapid response mechanism of the amygdala underscores its indispensable role in our survival, propelling swift actions that could mean the difference between safety and danger.

By understanding the amygdala's role like a security system, it becomes apparent why it is so crucial in managing how we react to the world around us, molding not only our immediate responses but also influencing our longer-term emotional health. With this in mind, appreciating the complexity and the quick-action efficiency of our brain's security guard brings a deeper understanding and appreciation of our intrinsic survival mechanisms.

Here is the detailed breakdown on the specific neural pathways, neurotransmitters, and biological reactions involved in the amygdala's response to threats, providing a clear understanding of our body's intrinsic 'security system':

- **Neural Pathways**:
    - **Pathway from Amygdala to Hypothalamus**: The amygdala sends signals directly to the hypothalamus, a critical area involved in activating the sympathetic nervous system, the system responsible for the 'fight-or-flight' response.
    - **Connection to the Sympathetic Nervous System**: From the hypothalamus, the activation pathway extends to

the spinal cord and then to various organs and muscles, preparing the body for rapid and intense physical activity.

- **Neurotransmitters Released**:
  - **Adrenaline (Epinephrine)**: Released primarily from the adrenal medulla (following signals from the sympathetic nervous system), adrenaline accelerates the heartbeat, increases breathing rate, and boosts energy production by stimulating glucose release. This prepares muscles for a burst of activity.
  - **Cortisol**: Cortisol, another stress hormone released during these times, increases sugars in the bloodstream and enhances the brain's use of glucose. It also curtails functions that would be nonessential or detrimental in a fight-or-flight situation.
  - **Norepinephrine**: Acts similarly to adrenaline but also sharpens focus, awareness, and responsiveness to sensory information, which is crucial when identifying and reacting to threats.

- **Biological Reactions**:
  - **Increase in Heart Rate**: The heart pumps faster to circulate blood more efficiently, delivering oxygen and nutrients to major muscle groups and vital organs faster.
  - **Heightened Senses**: Sensory systems become more acute, dilating pupils for better vision and sharpening hearing, essentially tuning all senses to detect and respond to the environment quickly.
  - **Muscle Preparation**: Blood flow to skeletal muscles increases, and muscles may tense up, priming the body for quick, powerful movements either to confront the danger or to flee from it.

Understanding these interactions and responses illuminates how the amygdala's activation, through a well-orchestrated series of neural and chemical events, equips us to deal with threats. This intricate system underscores not only our survival instincts but also demonstrates the complexity and efficiency of human physiology when faced with danger. By appreciating the functionality of these responses, individuals can better understand their own reactions to stress and fear, potentially guiding them toward more effective management of these instinctual responses in everyday life.

The prefrontal cortex serves as the cerebral embodiment of a wise counselor within our brains, moderating the impulses and primitive reactions initiated by other brain areas like the amygdala, notably during emotionally charged situations. It functions principally by applying a layer of rational thought to the raw, instinctive feelings generated when one confronts a provoking stimulus. This part of the brain assesses the longer-term consequences and social appropriateness of our initial emotional reactions, engaging in a complex decision-making process that often tempers impulsive behaviors.

For example, consider a scenario where an individual feels provoked by a comment during an important meeting. While the amygdala might trigger immediate feelings of anger or defensiveness, it's the prefrontal cortex that pauses to consider the implications of reacting angrily. It weighs the potential fallout from an outburst against the momentary satisfaction of retorting, potentially guiding the person to respond with calm and collected diplomacy instead.

By integrating past experiences and learned behaviors—such as the negative outcomes of previous angry outbursts—the prefrontal cortex helps to map out alternative responses. It enables us to take a breath, step back, and choose a course of action more aligned with our long-term objectives and social norms.

This moderating role of the prefrontal cortex is not just pivotal in managing emotional responses but is also crucial for planning complex cognitive behavior, personality expression, decision making, and moderating social behavior. By executing these functions, the prefrontal cortex helps us navigate our social world with greater finesse and maturity, adapting our responses to be as beneficial as possible both for immediate situations and for our broader life goals.

Hence, understanding how the prefrontal cortex operates to manage impulsive reactions is not just an academic exercise—it's directly applicable to enhancing personal and professional relationships, improving decision-making processes, and fostering more controlled and considered responses to emotional stimuli.

In understanding how our prefrontal cortex regulates emotions, it's crucial to follow the signals and processes involved in our brain's architecture. This step-by-step guide outlines the neurobiological pathways and mechanisms that govern emotional regulation.

Step 1: Neurological Pathways

The journey begins when an emotional stimulus is detected by the amygdala, the brain's alarm center for emotional processing. Upon detection, the amygdala sends urgent signals to the prefrontal cortex via the thalamus. This signal travels through a well-defined neural pathway known as the thalamo-cortical pathway. It's vital as it connects regions primarily responsible for emotional response and rational thinking.

Step 2: Neurotransmitter Actions

Once the signal reaches the prefrontal cortex, several neurotransmitters play key roles. Two pivotal ones include:

- **Serotonin**: Often dubbed the mood stabilizer, regulates mood, anxiety, and happiness. Higher levels generally improve one's ability to counteract the immediate, sometimes irrational, reactions triggered by the amygdala.

- **Dopamine**: Influences motivation and reward. It modulates the prefrontal cortex's activity by providing feedback about expected rewards or punishments, which helps in assessing whether an emotional reaction is worth the outcome.

Step 3: Decision-Making Process

With the data from neurotransmitters and the signal from the amygdala, the prefrontal cortex initiates a complex decision-making process:

- **Analysis**: First, it analyzes the emotional significance of the stimulus and recalls related past experiences from memory areas like the hippocampus.

- **Evaluation**: It then evaluates possible outcomes and consequences, weighing them against societal norms and personal values.

- **<u>Response Selection</u>**: Lastly, the prefrontal cortex chooses the most appropriate response, which could be to suppress an initial reaction or to take rational action based on logical deductions.

This cognitive appraisal and response modulation happen swiftly and are pivotal in managing how we react to everyday emotional stimulations. Understanding these steps helps clarify why sometimes we may feel overwhelmed but are able to respond appropriately, thanks to the moderating influence of the prefrontal cortex. This process is not just about controlling emotions but also about enhancing decision-making skills, ensuring that our responses are beneficial and aligned with long-term goals rather than just immediate, instinctual reactions.

Imagine the hippocampus as a meticulous librarian, not of books, but of your precious memories. Nestled deep within the brain, this librarian oversees a vast and intricate library where memories are cataloged and stored, mainly focusing on those imbued with emotional significance. Just as a librarian arranges books for efficient retrieval, the hippocampus organizes memory files based on emotional relevance, ensuring that some of your most vivid memories are accessible at a moment's notice.

When you encounter a situation that stirs emotions, it's like walking into the library and asking the librarian to pull out files related to similar past experiences. For instance, the smell of a specific perfume might transport you back to a significant moment in your life, because the hippocampus has efficiently linked that scent to a powerful, emotional memory, just as a librarian might find a note tucked within a favorite book.

This isn't just about storing memories; it's about enhancing our understanding of the world. By sorting these emotional memories, the hippocampus allows us to react appropriately to new experiences based on past lessons. It connects threads of past emotions and events to present situations, helping guide our responses—a form of emotional intelligence that is crucial for navigating complex social interactions.

Recognizing the role of the hippocampus as our brain's "librarian" not only clarifies how memory works but also underscores the profound impact that our stored experiences have on our daily lives. It highlights why certain memories pop up unexpectedly and how our emotional landscape shapes our perception of the world. This understanding doesn't just enrich our knowledge of brain function; it connects deeply to our personal and emotional growth.

Here is the breakdown on the neurobiology of memory formation and retrieval in the hippocampus, specifically focusing on the encoding and recall of emotional memories:

- **Memory Encoding**:
    - Emotional experiences are translated into lasting memory traces in the hippocampus. This process begins when an emotional event activates a network of neurons that

represent various aspects of the experience (sensory, cognitive, emotional).

- Neurochemical and hormonal systems, particularly those activated during emotional arousal, enhance memory encoding by modifying the strength of the synaptic connections between these neurons.

- **Neural Pathways**:
- **Sensory Input to Encoding**: Information from sensory organs is relayed to the amygdala and other sensory processing areas in the cortex, then transmitted to the hippocampus. This pathway is crucial as it helps to link external stimuli with appropriate emotional responses.
- **Integration**: The hippocampus integrates this sensory information with cognitive data from the cortex, forming a coherent memory trace that encompasses both the factual and emotional aspects of the memory.

- **Memory Retrieval**:
- Retrieval of emotional memories is facilitated when similar sensory or emotional conditions are present. The hippocampus accesses and reactivates the neural circuits originally involved in encoding the memory.
- This reactivation process helps to bring the memory into conscious awareness, often with vivid emotional and sensory detail, due to the strong connections formed during the initial encoding.

- **Role of Neurotransmitters**:
- **Glutamate**: The primary excitatory neurotransmitter in the brain, glutamate facilitates the formation of new

memories by enhancing synaptic plasticity and neural connectivity in the hippocampus.

- **GABA**: As the main inhibitory neurotransmitter, GABA helps to regulate memory encoding and retrieval by balancing the excitatory signals mediated by glutamate, ensuring that the hippocampus does not become overstimulated.

- **Dopamine and Norepinephrine**: Released in response to emotionally charged events, these neurotransmitters enhance the encoding of emotional memories by increasing attention and enhancing the consolidation of information into long-term memory storage.

This detailed exploration into the mechanisms of memory processing in the hippocampus elucidates how emotionally charged experiences are imprinted, stored, and recalled. Understanding these processes underscores the powerful influence of emotional contexts on our memory systems and highlights the intricate ways our brains manage and utilize memories to navigate the world.

Grasping the neural underpinnings of emotions is more than an academic exercise; it offers profound practical benefits in enhancing emotional intelligence, boosting mental health, and improving interpersonal relationships. The brain's intricate network governs how emotions are experienced and regulated, directly influencing behavior and interactions with others.

Starting with emotional intelligence, understanding the mechanisms of emotional processing—such as how the amygdala reacts to threats or how the prefrontal cortex moderates responses—can improve one's ability to monitor personal and others' emotions. For instance, recognizing when the amygdala triggers a fight-or-flight response can help someone identify feelings of anxiety or anger quickly. This awareness can lead to more effective strategies for managing those emotions, such as deep breathing or cognitive reappraisal, enhancing personal well-being.

In terms of mental health, knowledge of the brain's emotional pathways aids in identifying dysfunctions which may lead to mental illnesses. For instance, an overactive amygdala might be linked to heightened anxiety. Therapists often use this information to design targeted treatments such as Psychotherapy or mindfulness techniques, which can help recalibrate the emotional responses by practicing new thinking patterns and behaviors.

Regarding interpersonal relationships, an understanding of emotional brain function allows for empathy—a foundational element of social interaction. By realizing that emotions can cloud judgment or trigger defensive reactions, one can learn to respond rather than react during heated discussions with friends, family, or colleagues. For example, understanding that a partner's sharp reaction might stem from a stress-triggered amygdala response can foster patience and support rather than conflict.

Therefore, diving deep into the brain's role in emotional dynamics not only enriches one's understanding of human psychology but also equips individuals with tools to navigate the complexities of emotions in their personal and social lives. This knowledge empowers one to lead a more emotionally intelligent, mentally healthy, and socially connected life.

Let's take a deeper look at the neurophysiological processes involved in emotional regulation, examining the intricate journey from perception to reaction, and how this influences behavior in real-life situations.

Detailed Neural Pathways:
The process begins when an emotional stimulus is perceived—say, a startling noise or a stressful interaction. Sensory receptors send this information directly to the thalamus, which acts as the brain's relay station. The thalamus then forwards these signals to two key brain areas: the amygdala and the prefrontal cortex.
 - **Amygdala**: Known as the emotional center of the brain, the amygdala assesses the emotional significance of the stimulus and prepares an immediate response. This reaction is quick and visceral, often activating before the conscious mind has fully processed the information.
 - **Prefrontal Cortex**: Acting as a moderator, the prefrontal cortex receives the initial reactions from the amygdala and begins the regulation process. It evaluates the appropriateness of the response based on past experiences, predicted future outcomes, and current social norms, potentially dampening or enhancing the amygdala's raw response.

Neurotransmitter Functions:
Neurotransmitters play critical roles in how these signals

are modulated and interpreted.

- **Serotonin**: Often associated with mood regulation, serotonin levels influence how emotional responses are processed in the prefrontal cortex. Higher serotonin levels generally help promote a more balanced, calm reaction to stress.

- **Dopamine**: Dopamine is tied to reward and motivation circuits. In the context of emotional regulation, dopamine can amplify the perception of emotional stimuli, affecting how intensely an individual reacts to positive or negative events.

- **GABA**: As the brain's primary inhibitory neurotransmitter, GABA helps reduce neuronal excitability throughout the nervous system, including in the amygdala, thereby playing a key role in calming down immediate emotional responses.

Behavioral Outputs:

The culmination of these processes results in observable behaviors that manifest physically and psychologically.

- **Stress Reaction**: In a stress response facilitated by low serotonin and high amygdala activity, an individual might experience increased heart rate, sweating, and anxiety—clear physical manifestations.

- **Calmness in Interactions**: With effective prefrontal regulation and balanced neurotransmitter activity, a person may exhibit calmness and control in potentially heated interactions, able to respond thoughtfully rather than react impulsively.

Understanding these detailed neurophysiological mechanisms provides valuable insights into the basis of emotional responses and offers strategies for managing them more effectively. By recognizing what's happening inside the brain during emotional events, individuals can better regulate their responses to align with desired outcomes in personal and professional realms, enhancing emotional intelligence and improving overall mental well-being. This knowledge not only empowers us to handle our emotions more effectively but also improves our interactions and relationships, enriching our lives and the lives of those around us.

Our exploration of the brain's emotional landscape reveals a complex network where feelings are not just ephemeral states but deeply integrated processes influenced by various brain structures like the amygdala, hippocampus, and prefrontal cortex. This understanding provides us with a clearer lens through which we can view our emotional reactions and behaviors. It emphasizes how our daily experiences and interactions are profoundly shaped by the intricate workings of our brain.

Recognizing the role of these neural substrates in emotional regulation not only enriches our knowledge but also underscores the importance of ongoing education and personal mindfulness. By continuing to learn about the neurological underpinnings of emotions, we equip ourselves with the tools necessary to enhance our emotional intelligence, manage stress more effectively, and improve our relationships with others.

The journey through the brain's emotional pathways is an ongoing process of discovery and adaptation. With each piece of new knowledge, we gather insights that can lead to more mindful responses and healthier emotional engagements in our lives. Thus, fostering a habit of continuous learning and self-awareness is crucial for anyone looking to navigate the complexities of emotions with more grace and effectiveness. By committing to this educational pursuit, each individual gains the opportunity to lead a more balanced and fulfilling emotional life.

SENSORY AND MOTOR PATHWAYS

In the intricate dance of human interaction with the world, sensory and motor pathways play a pivotal role, allowing us to understand and respond appropriately to our environment. These biological highways carry information from every corner of our bodies to the brain, where it's processed, and then deliver commands back to our muscles, guiding them in a coordinated ballet of responses. This dynamic flow underpins every action, from the simple act of blinking to the complex maneuvers of an athlete.

Understanding how these pathways work is essential for appreciating the elegance and efficiency with which our bodies navigate daily tasks. It offers insights into everything from why we jerk our hands away from a hot stove, to how we can drive cars or play pianos—activities that demand rapid, precise interactions between sensory inputs and motor outputs. This chapter walks you through the biology of these pathways, explaining how they maintain seamless communication between the brain and body, ensuring we can move, react, and interact with the world around us effectively.

Far from being just a subject of scientific curiosity, the knowledge of these pathways enriches our understanding of human capability and resilience, providing a clearer picture of how we adapt to and influence our surroundings. By diving into the mechanics of these extraordinary systems, we not only gain a deeper respect for the human body's complexity but also open doors to enhancing our interaction with the external world through advances in technology and healthcare.

Sensory pathways are crucial networks within the body that transport information from sensory receptors to the brain. These receptors, which are located throughout the body, detect changes in the environment such as heat, light, pressure, and chemicals, and convert these changes into electrical signals. The journey of these signals begins at the receptor sites, where a specific stimulus—like the heat from a stove or the coolness of a breeze—triggers a response.

Once activated, these electrical signals travel through neurons, the specialized cells responsible for carrying information. The first neuron in this pathway transmits the signal to a relay station in the central nervous system, typically the spinal cord or directly to the brain stem. Here, the signal might be refined or modulated to ensure the brain receives accurate information.

The relay station then sends the signal upwards to different areas of the brain, including the thalamus, which acts as a central hub for processing. The thalamus filters out unnecessary noise and emphasizes essential signals based on the current focus and needs of the body. After processing in the thalamus, the information is forwarded to the cerebral cortex, the area of the brain that interprets the signal and formulates an appropriate response. For example, if you touch a hot surface, the sensory pathways alert the brain about the high temperature, and almost instantaneously, the brain processes this and sends a command back through motor pathways to pull your hand away, often before you even consciously register the burn.

Understanding the structure and operations of sensory pathways not only allows us to grasp how we interact seamlessly with our environment but also helps in diagnosing and treating sensory disorders. By mapping out these neural highways, scientists and doctors can better understand where interruptions in these pathways might lead to sensory impairments, enhancing our ability to address such challenges effectively. Thus, the study of sensory pathways not only feeds our curiosity about human biology but also holds practical implications for improving health and well-being.

Let's take a deeper look at how sensory pathways convert environmental stimuli into neural messages that our brain can understand, following the path from the molecular mechanisms at sensory receptors through sophisticated processing in the thalamus.

- **<u>Signal Transduction at Receptors</u>**: At the molecular level, sensory receptors—specialized proteins or cells located at the terminal ends of sensory neurons—detect specific types of stimuli. For heat, thermoreceptors respond by changing their structure as temperatures rise or fall, altering ion permeability and generating electrical signals. Photoreceptors in the eye convert light into electrical signals through a process where light changes the shape of the protein rhodopsin, initiating a cascade that results in the closure of ion channels. Mechanoreceptors respond to physical pressure by opening ion channels directly in response to the mechanical deformation of the receptor cell's membrane.

- **Types of Sensory Neurons**: There are several types of sensory neurons, which can be distinguished by their structure, location, and the type of stimuli they detect. For instance:
    - **Pseudounipolar neurons**: Found in the dorsal root ganglia of the spinal cord, these neurons have a single process that splits into two branches; one connecting to the periphery and the other entering the spinal cord, ideal for transmitting sensory information.
    - **Bipolar neurons**: Commonly found in the retina of the eye, these neurons have one axon and one dendrite and are crucial in the process of visual transduction.

- **Neurotransmitter Actions at Relay Stations**: Within relay stations like the spinal cord and brain stem, neurotransmitters play key roles in modulating sensory inputs. For example, glutamate is often released by sensory neurons to excite neurons in the spinal cord, which then sends the signals up to the brain. On the other hand, inhibitory neurotransmitters like GABA are released to prevent over-excitation and to refine the sensory input, ensuring that only relevant signals are intensified.

- **Thalamus Processing**: The thalamus acts as a crucial relay and processing station within the brain. Each region of the thalamus is connected to specific areas of the cortex and other parts of the brain, integrating sensory messages. Here, the thalamus filters incoming signals, prioritizing them based on factors such as intensity and relevance to current activities. This filtering is achieved through a mix of synaptic connections and neurotransmitter actions, which either amplify key signals or dampen background noise, ensuring that the cerebral cortex receives data that is most pertinent for immediate decision-making and response.

Understanding these intricate processes underscores the precision with which our nervous system operates, enabling timely and appropriate responses to our environment. By appreciating the close interaction between various neuronal types and molecular mechanisms, one gains a richer understanding of how our sensory experiences are constructed, leading to insights that are not only fascinating but also critical for fields ranging from neuroscience to medicine.

Motor pathways in the human body are essential circuits responsible for controlling both voluntary and involuntary movements. These pathways originate in the brain's motor cortex, where decisions about movement are made and signals are sent through the spinal cord to various muscles. In voluntary movements, such as reaching out to shake a hand or writing with a pen, these pathways enable precise and conscious control over muscle groups. The sensory inputs, like the texture of the pen or the sight of a hand extending for a shake, inform the brain which then sends specific instructions back through these motor pathways to achieve the desired action.

In contrast, involuntary movements are those that occur

without conscious decision, primarily involving reflexes and automatic responses such as pulling a hand back from a hot surface. These movements are facilitated by motor pathways that bypass higher conscious areas of the brain, enabling faster responses critical for safety and basic physiological functions.

An example illustrating the significance of these pathways occurs in sports, where an athlete like a basketball player must combine voluntary movements (aiming for a shot) with involuntary reflexes (reacting to an unexpected pass). The motor pathways coordinate these complex tasks by rapidly processing neural signals and issuing commands to the muscles.

Understanding the functions and operations of motor pathways not only provides insight into basic human actions but is critical in addressing motor control issues arising from neurological disorders. In conditions where these pathways are damaged, such as in stroke or spinal cord injuries, regaining motor function involves retraining these pathways, often utilizing therapies that stimulate both voluntary and involuntary movement processes.

By studying motor pathways, we gain insights crucial for medical rehabilitation techniques, enhancing athletic training and improving our overall understanding of human biomechanics. This knowledge propels advancements in medical technology and therapeutic practices, ultimately improving the quality of life for individuals impacted by motor function impairments.

Let's take a deeper look at the complex interplay of neuroanatomical structures, neurochemical processes, and innovative recovery therapies that underpin motor pathway functions and contribute to motion control and rehabilitation after injuries.

- **Neuroanatomical Structures**: The motor cortex, located in the frontal lobe of the brain, plays a pivotal role in motor control. It's divided into the primary motor cortex, premotor cortex, and supplementary motor area, each contributing uniquely to movement. The primary motor cortex directly sends signals to motor neurons in the spinal cord, which then connect to muscle fibers to execute movement. The premotor cortex assists in planning movements, and the supplementary motor area coordinates movements involving both limbs simultaneously. Together, these areas form a precise network that directs voluntary muscular activity.

- **Neurochemical Processes**: Neurotransmitters are crucial in facilitating the transmission of motor commands across synapses. Acetylcholine is a key neurotransmitter at neuromuscular junctions, where nerve impulses are converted into actions in muscle fibers. In the central nervous system, neurotransmitters like glutamate play a major role in promoting excitatory signals that activate motor neurons, while GABA and glycine typically serve inhibitory functions, preventing excessive movement and ensuring coordination.

- **Recovery Therapies**: Modern medicine offers several therapeutic approaches to restore motor function following neural damage. Neuroplasticity-promoting practices, such as constraint-induced movement therapy, are designed to engage the brain's natural ability to reorganize and form new neural connections. Electrical stimulation therapies like Functional Electrical Stimulation (FES) help restore movement to paralyzed muscles by applying small electrical pulses to weakened or atrophied muscles. Furthermore, robotic-assisted therapies provide repetitive motion practice to aid the recovery of limb functions, which is crucial after events like a stroke or spinal cord injury.

Each of these components—from the detailed workings of the motor cortex to the advanced recovery therapies—plays a significant role in how humans control movements and recover from motor impairments. By unraveling these complexities, we not only gain insights into the fundamental operations of our own bodies but also pave the way for innovative treatments and improved life quality for those affected by motor function challenges. This knowledge arms clinicians, therapists, and patients with the tools to better manage and potentially overcome the limitations imposed by neurological conditions.

The neural circuits responsible for sensory perception and motor control are intricately designed to process and respond to environmental stimuli swiftly and effectively. These circuits begin with sensory receptors located throughout the body, which detect changes in the environment, such as touch, temperature, and sound. Each receptor type is specialized to convert specific physical or chemical stimuli into electrical signals, which are then relayed to the brain through dedicated sensory neurons.

Upon reaching the brain, these signals enter the thalamus, which acts as a central relay station. The thalamus filters and directs sensory information to appropriate areas of the cerebral cortex, where sensory inputs are interpreted as perceptions. This integration enables the brain to construct a coherent picture of the surrounding environment, informing subsequent decisions and responses.

For motor control, the process initiates in the motor areas of the cerebral cortex, where the planning, control, and execution of voluntary movements occur. The primary motor cortex generates neural impulses that travel down the spinal cord to motor neurons, which directly innervate muscles. The precise coordination and timing of these signals are critical for smooth and purposeful movement.

The cerebellum and basal ganglia support these processes by regulating the balance, coordination, and fine-tuning of movements, ensuring that responses are not only rapid but also appropriately adapted to the context. For instance, catching a swiftly thrown ball requires rapid sensory processing to track the ball's path and equally quick motor responses to position the hands correctly.

This neural orchestration allows for the seamless execution of complex tasks, from the simple act of swatting away a fly to the intricate maneuvers involved in driving a car through traffic. The efficiency and adaptability of these neural circuits underscore their evolutionary importance, enabling humans to navigate and interact with a dynamic and sometimes unpredictable environment effectively.

Understanding these pathways not only fascinates those curious about human biology but also has practical implications in areas like neurorehabilitation and robotics, where mimicking or repairing these natural processes can significantly improve lives. This knowledge empowers us to appreciate the underlying biological mechanisms that drive our interactions with the world, providing a deeper insight into both the capabilities and vulnerabilities of the human body.

In the thalamus, synaptic mechanisms play a crucial role in processing sensory information before it reaches the cerebral cortex. As sensory signals arrive, they are subject to both enhancement and inhibition through synaptic activities. Neurotransmitters like glutamate and GABA dictate these processes. Glutamate acts to excite neurons, amplifying relevant sensory data to ensure the cortex receives distinct and necessary signals for accurate perception. Conversely, GABA serves as an inhibitory messenger, helping to dampen any excessive noise in the signal, thus preventing overload and potential confusion in the cortical response.

Moving to the motor cortex, the array of neurotransmitters orchestrating movement is equally intricate. Here, the principal neurotransmitter is acetylcholine, which carries signals from neurons in the motor cortex directly to motor neurons in the spinal cord and muscles. This neurotransmission is vital for the initiation and modulation of voluntary movements. The precise release of acetylcholine at synaptic junctions ensures that motor commands are effectively communicated to muscles, resulting in coordinated motion.

Neural plasticity in these pathways allows for the extraordinary capability to adapt to a changing environment. Through a process known as synaptic plasticity, neurons can strengthen or weaken their connections based on activity levels. This adaptive mechanism is key for both sensory and motor systems. In sensory pathways, it enables heightened sensitivity or desensitization to particular stimuli based on their relevance or frequency. In motor pathways, plasticity facilitates the refinement of movements, improving coordination and skill over time as one repeatedly practices an activity.

These detailed molecular interactions and synaptic activities form the foundation of how humans perceive and interact with the world. Understanding these mechanisms provides deeper insights into the functioning of our nervous system, highlighting the sophisticated nature of our interactions with our environment and the capacity for learning and adaptation that defines human experience.

Imagine the interactions between sensory inputs and motor outputs as a bustling city traffic system. In this city, the sensory inputs are like the myriad vehicles that bring information from all over—the sights, sounds, and smells are collected from various sources, such as cars, bikes, and pedestrians arriving from suburban areas to the central hub. This hub can be likened to the brain's thalamus, a major interchange where all sensory data is assessed and directed.

Signals that pass through the thalamus are like cars being routed to different parts of the city, making sure that all the information reaches the right destinations. These destinations, the cerebral cortex areas, resemble different neighborhoods that specialize in various functions—like a district for arts where visuals are processed, an industrial zone for sounds, and a culinary quarter for smells and tastes.

Once these neighborhoods process the incoming data, they need to respond—here's where motor outputs come into play. Think of them as service vehicles that carry out the necessary actions based on the information processed. If a neighborhood reports a fire, the motor outputs are the fire trucks leaving the central fire station—the motor cortex—rushing down the spinal cord highway to reach the muscles that act as firefighters to extinguish the blaze by pulling a hand back from a hot object.

This entire operational system ensures that the city functions smoothly, handling incoming information, processing it, and responding appropriately through a well-organized network of roads, vehicles, and services. Just as a city planner would optimize traffic flow and emergency responses, the human body fine-tunes its neural pathways for sensory perception and motor control to interact effectively with the environment, showcasing a sophisticated blend of biology and functionality similar to urban planning. This not only illustrates the complexity of our neural functions but also underscores their importance in our daily navigation and survival in the dynamic world around us.

Here is the detailed breakdown on the various types of sensory inputs and the intricacies of signal processing within the neural pathways:

- **Types of Sensory Inputs**:
  - **Tactile (Touch)**: Detected by mechanoreceptors in the skin, which respond to different stimuli such as pressure, vibration, and texture. The initial neural response involves the conversion of mechanical stimulus into an electrical signal, which is then transmitted via sensory neurons to the spinal cord and brain.
  - **Auditory (Sound)**: Sound waves are captured by the ear and translated into mechanical vibrations by the eardrum. These vibrations are converted into electrical signals in the cochlea through hair cells. The signals are then sent through the auditory nerve to the brain.
  - **Visual (Sight)**: Light enters the eye, focusing on the retina, where photoreceptors (rods and cones) convert light into electrical signals. These signals travel from the retina through the optic nerve to the brain.
  - **Olfactory (Smell)**: Odor molecules bind to receptors in the olfactory epithelium in the nose, initiating a neural response that transmits signals to the olfactory bulb and then to the brain, enabling scent perception.

- **Signal Processing from Thalamus to Cerebral Cortex**:
  - **Neurological Pathways**: Once sensory signals reach the thalamus, they are relayed to specific regions of the cerebral cortex dedicated to processing each type of sensory input. For instance, visual signals are sent to the visual cortex, auditory signals to the auditory cortex, and so on.

- **Signal Filtering and Prioritization**: In the thalamus, sensory information undergoes significant processing. Signals are filtered to reduce redundancy, enhance signal-to-noise ratio, and prioritize based on current attentional focus and relevance to ongoing activities. For example, in a dangerous situation, the sounds of approaching vehicles might be prioritized over less critical sounds.

- **Enhancement of Signals**: The thalamus also plays a role in enhancing signals that are deemed important. This involves amplifying neural responses to ensure that vital information is perceived more distinctly, facilitating quicker and more appropriate behavioral responses.

This comprehensive view of sensory processing illuminates how different stimuli are detected, processed, and integrated to produce coherent and timely responses that enable individuals to navigate and interact effectively with their environment. Understanding these processes highlights the sophistication of the neural systems and underscores the critical role of sensory perception in everyday life.

Understanding sensory and motor pathways is pivotal in advancing prosthetic and robotic technologies that either mimic or enhance natural body functions. Deep insights into how these pathways function provide critical data that engineers use to create devices that interact seamlessly with the human body. One core aspect is the development of prosthetic limbs that not only replicate movements but also provide sensory feedback similar to natural limbs. For instance, sensors on a prosthetic hand can detect tactile information, like pressure and temperature, and convert these into electrical signals that stimulate the wearer's nerve endings, allowing the person to 'feel' the object.

Moreover, the knowledge of motor pathways drives the integration of muscle signals to control these prosthetics. Techniques like targeted muscle reinnervation redirect amputated nerves to remaining muscles, which then behave as control sites for the prosthetic limbs based on the signals they receive, which were originally intended for the missing limb. This allows for more intuitive control of the prosthetics, closely mimicking natural motor responses.

In the realm of robotics, understanding these pathways helps in designing more efficient and adaptable robots that can perform complex human-like tasks independently. Robots equipped with AI that mimics human sensory and motor processing can interact in more nuanced and contextually appropriate ways, improving their functionality in diverse environments, from factories to homes.

The influence of this technology extends beyond mere replacement or enhancement of physical abilities — it fundamentally improves the quality of life, providing independence and increased capabilities. For individuals with disabilities, such advancements are not just technological improvements but gateways to enhanced mobility, interaction, and personal freedom.

By continuing to explore and understand the intricate details of sensory and motor pathways, researchers can further refine these technologies, making them more accessible and adaptable to a wider range of needs. This ongoing progress not only showcases the marvel of human ingenuity but also aligns closely with our innate understanding of movement and interaction, marking a significant leap in how humans interface with technology.

In the realm of robotics, Artificial Intelligence (AI) plays a pivotal role in mimicking human sensory and motor functions, propelling robots from mere machines to adaptive and responsive entities. Here's a detailed guide on how AI integrates and operates within robotic systems:

1. **AI Algorithms in Robotics**:
   - **Types of AI Algorithms**: Robots utilize a variety of AI algorithms, including neural networks, machine learning, and deep learning. These algorithms enable robots to emulate human perception and movement.
   - **Interpreting Sensory Data**: AI systems analyze inputs from sensors (similar to human senses) using convolutional neural networks (CNNs). For instance, in visual processing, CNNs can identify and categorize objects within the robot's field of view, mimicking human visual recognition.
   - **Decision-Making and Motor Control**: Once data is interpreted, decision-making algorithms assess the best response. This involves planning algorithms like Dijkstra's or A* for navigating space, or reinforcement learning for adapting strategies based on previous outcomes. The selected response is translated into motor commands that control the robot's actuators.

2. **Integration of Sensory Data**:
   - **Processing Complex Data**: AI systems merge data from various sensors to form a unified model of the environment. This multisensory integration is crucial for robots to function in a human-like manner, providing a holistic view and situational awareness.
   - **Contextual Decision-Making**: Advanced AI models, incorporating elements of predictive analytics, evaluate not just current sensory inputs but also predict potential future states. This allows robots to make proactive decisions, such as a robot in a manufacturing plant slowing down operations after detecting signs of wear in equipment.

3. **Motor Control Through AI**:
   - **Interpreting Commands**: AI interfaces interpret high-level goals into specific motor commands. For instance, if the goal is to grasp an object, the AI calculates the trajectory, force, and finger positions needed, translating these into commands for the robotic arm's motors.
   - **Real-Time Adaptation**: Robots equipped with AI adjust their actions in real-time using feedback loops from sensors. If a robot's arm encounters unexpected resistance while lifting an object, sensors detect the change, and the AI adjusts the motor output to compensate—similar to how humans apply more force when lifting a heavier-than-expected object.

This granular view of AI in robotic systems illustrates not only how robots can replicate human sensory and motor activities but also enhance their functionalities for efficiency and adaptability. As AI algorithms and sensory technologies continue to evolve, the integration and responsiveness of these robotic systems will increasingly converge with human-like capabilities, making them indispensable in diverse settings from industries to homes. This symbiotic relationship between AI and robotics heralds a future where robots are not just tools, but partners in everyday human activities.

This chapter has comprehensively examined how sensory and motor pathways operate within the human body, demonstrating their critical roles in both our daily activities and complex behaviors. It has shown that these pathways are not just pathways for nerve impulses but intricate networks that enable us to perceive, interact with, and respond to our environment efficiently. The discussion highlighted technological advancements in prosthetics and robotics as direct applications of our growing understanding of these neural paths.

As research continues to peel back layers of complexity in sensory and motor pathways, the potential for future scientific and medical innovations seems boundless. Enhanced comprehension could lead to more sophisticated neural prostheses that offer improved integration and functionality, closely mirroring natural human abilities. In medicine, insights into these pathways may pave the way for novel treatments for neurological disorders, potentially offering improved outcomes for conditions that affect motor skills and sensory perception.

Diving even deeper, the ongoing exploration of how these pathways work at molecular and genetic levels could revolutionize our approach to preventive medicine. By understanding the building blocks of sensory and motor functions, we could foresee and intercept dysfunctions before they manifest into more severe conditions. The journey of discovery in this field is ongoing, promising not only to expand our knowledge but also to enhance the quality of life in tangible ways. Through continued research and technological integration, the future of how we understand and interact with our biological systems holds unprecedented potential.

THE DEVELOPING BRAIN

The human brain, a masterful orchestrator of thought, emotion, and behavior, undergoes an extraordinary transformation from infancy through adulthood. This chapter, "The Developing Brain," unpacks the intricate journey of how the brain evolves, focusing on crucial developmental stages that mark both physical growth and cognitive enhancement. Here, we explore the continuous and dynamic process of brain development which shapes our entire being—understanding how a mere cluster of cells in an embryo blossoms into a complex organ capable of profound thoughts and emotions.

From the synaptic exuberance of early childhood, where the brain's plasticity allows for rapid learning and adaptability, to the refinement and consolidation seen in adult years, each stage of brain development offers new insights into the foundations of human nature. As we delve into the layers of neural pathways and their maturation, we see how these transformations relate directly to changes in behavior and mental capabilities.

With clarity and precision, we will navigate these developmental milestones, shedding light on how each phase not only contributes to who we are but also impacts our lifelong learning and mental health. Through the lenses of modern science and poignant examples, this chapter aims not just to inform but to enrich your understanding of the ever-evolving human brain. It's a testament to the remarkable capabilities inherent within us and a nod to the potential that future scientific and medical advancements hold in harnessing this knowledge for better health outcomes.

Neural plasticity, particularly vigorous during early childhood, is the brain's ability to reorganize itself by forming new neural connections. This flexibility allows the brain to adapt to new experiences, learn, and memorize by strengthening the synapses—a process essential in the early stages of cognitive and behavioral development. During these formative years, the brain's plastic nature means it is exceptionally receptive to the learning that comes from sensory experiences, whether tactile, visual, auditory, or social.

For instance, consider the way language skills develop in young children—a direct consequence of neural plasticity. Exposed to language, a child's brain rapidly creates and strengthens neural pathways associated with the sounds and meanings of words. This is why children who grow up in bilingual environments often excel at both languages from a young age—they are leveraging the heightened plasticity of their developing brains to wire pathways for two linguistic systems simultaneously.

Another compelling example is the impact of musical training during early childhood. Studies have shown that children who engage in regular musical practice experience significant enhancements in areas of the brain responsible for audio processing and motor control, comparatively more than those who do not participate in such activities. This is because the repeated practice and sensory input from musical activities exploit the brain's plasticity, fostering cognitive and motor skills that benefit children across multiple domains, including academic performance and social interactions.

This detailed look at neural plasticity underscores its pivotal role in shaping a child's intellectual and emotional landscape. As we continue to explore how various stimuli influence early brain development, it becomes increasingly clear that the experiences children undergo in their formative years have lasting impacts, sculpting their cognitive abilities and behavioral patterns in profound ways. This understanding not only enlightens current educational and parenting practices but also encourages a nurturing environment that can significantly enhance a child's development through carefully chosen experiences and interactions.

Let's take a closer look at the intricate biochemical processes that underpin synapse strengthening during the critical phase of early childhood neural plasticity.

Synaptic Strengthening Mechanisms:

At the heart of synaptic strengthening is a biochemical process known as Long-Term Potentiation (LTP). This process primarily involves the neurotransmitter glutamate, which plays a pivotal role in enhancing synaptic efficacy. When a synapse is repeatedly activated, glutamate is released into the synaptic cleft and binds to receptors on the post-synaptic neuron, such as NMDA (N-methyl-D-aspartate) and AMPA (α-amino-3-hydroxy-5-methyl-4-isoxazolepropionic acid) receptors. The activation of NMDA receptors leads to an influx of calcium ions into the neuron, which triggers a cascade of intracellular events that ultimately strengthen the synapse by increasing the sensitivity and number of AMPA receptors, thereby enhancing synaptic transmission.

Neurotransmitter Roles:

Various neurotransmitters are involved in early childhood learning and memory formation, each playing a unique role in the brain's development. Beyond glutamate, neurotransmitters like dopamine and acetylcholine are crucial for reinforcing learning and memory. Dopamine modulation influences reward-related learning, which helps children associate certain behaviors with positive outcomes. Acetylcholine enhances attention and arousal, facilitating the encoding of new memories during learning processes. Their interaction with specific receptors activates signal transduction pathways that lead to transcriptional changes and structural modifications in neural circuits, supporting cognitive development.

Impact of External Stimuli:

External stimuli such as auditory and tactile inputs play a significant role in triggering these molecular events. For example, when a child is repeatedly exposed to language sounds, the auditory cortex becomes activated, utilizing mechanisms of LTP to enhance the efficiency of sound processing pathways. Similarly, tactile inputs from activities like handling musical instruments prompt specific regions in the somatosensory cortex to adapt and refine their synaptic connections. These experiences lead to the preferential strengthening of neural pathways that are frequently used, which is a fundamental aspect of neural plasticity.

Understanding these biochemical details not only sheds light on the complexity and adaptability of the developing brain but also emphasizes the critical importance of providing stimulating and enriching environments for children. This knowledge underscores how tailored educational strategies can significantly impact cognitive and emotional development, ultimately enhancing learning outcomes and personal growth.

Critical periods in brain development refer to specific phases during which the brain is exceptionally responsive to certain environmental stimuli, making these windows crucial for acquiring particular skills or behaviors. This concept has profound implications for language acquisition and emotional development, as these periods define the optimal times for learning languages and forming key emotional capacities.

For instance, the critical period for language acquisition typically peaks before puberty. During this time, the neural circuitry for language is especially plastic, facilitating the absorption of linguistic nuances that become harder to master as one ages. Notable examples include linguist Noam Chomsky, whose theories of language acquisition suggest that children are born with an innate ability to learn language. This premise is supported by observing children who grow up in multilingual environments, such as novelist Jhumpa Lahiri, who proficiently mastered multiple languages early in life, undoubtedly influenced by her exposure during this critical window.

Similarly, emotional development is deeply tied to critical periods during which children are particularly sensitive to social and emotional cues. This sensitivity helps in forming secure attachments and in developing complex emotional understanding. Psychologist John Bowlby's attachment theory underscores the importance of supportive care during the early years, which impacts individuals' emotional health throughout life. An exemplary case is that of Tenzin Gyatso, the 14th Dalai Lama, whose early teachings on compassion and mindfulness have portrayed profound emotional awareness and intelligence.

These examples underscore the necessity of maximizing the learning and developmental potential available during these critical periods. By understanding and aligning educational and parenting approaches to these timeframes, one can significantly influence a child's linguistic abilities and emotional health, providing a robust foundation for later success. This knowledge not only enriches individual lives but also informs broader educational and social policies aimed at nurturing well-rounded, emotionally intelligent individuals.

Let's take a deeper look at the complex neurological processes during critical periods of brain development, and how they interact with environmental stimuli to shape our cognitive and emotional capabilities.

Neurological Underpinnings:

During critical periods, certain brain structures and neuronal processes exhibit heightened malleability, making them especially receptive to external influences. Key areas like the auditory cortex for language or the limbic system for emotional processing are primed for rapid development. Synaptic plasticity, the brain's ability to strengthen or weaken synapses based on activity, plays a fundamental role in this phase. Additionally, neurogenesis—the creation of new neurons—continues at a remarkable rate, particularly in regions like the hippocampus, which is central to learning and memory. These processes ensure that the brain's architecture can adapt quickly and effectively to new information.

Environmental Interaction:

Environmental stimuli critically interact with these malleable brain structures to guide development. For example, language exposure during early childhood triggers activity in the language-related regions of the brain, which rely on synaptic plasticity to fine-tune the neural circuits necessary for language comprehension and speech. Emotional interactions, on the other hand, engage the limbic system; nurturing care can foster strong synaptic connections that support emotional stability and resilience. Both chemical messengers, like neurotransmitters, and physical changes in synaptic strength, facilitate these adaptations, directly impacting the brain's developmental trajectory.

Implication on Development:

These neuro-environmental interactions are instrumental

in forming complex linguistic structures and sophisticated emotional responses. For instance, children exposed to multiple languages often develop a more nuanced linguistic framework, as their brain capitalizes on synaptic plasticity to accommodate and separate different linguistic systems. Emotionally, children who receive consistent and empathetic interaction may develop more robust neural pathways that support healthy emotional expressions and relationships. Enhanced synaptic connections in response to these stimuli not only shape immediate behaviors and skills but also set foundational patterns that influence long-term cognitive and emotional health.

Understanding these intricate interactions during critical developmental windows offers profound insights into the dynamic interplay between nature and nurture in shaping human development. By fostering environments that align with the neurological needs of critical development periods, we can greatly enhance educational outcomes and emotional well-being, paving the way for individuals to reach their full potential in all aspects of life.

Imagine your brain as a bustling garden during adolescence, where the process of synaptic pruning perfectly mirrors the attentive work of a seasoned gardener. In this vibrant garden, the brain's synapses are like the myriad of branches on numerous lush plants. During the early years of life, just as a gardener might initially allow plants to grow wildly to see which are strongest, the brain forms an abundance of synapses more than necessary.

As adolescence arrives, similar to the gardener deciding

it's time to optimize the garden's health and aesthetics, the brain begins the crucial process of synaptic pruning. The gardener evaluates each plant, trimming away weaker or less necessary branches, allowing the stronger and more essential ones to flourish. Similarly, the brain, throughout adolescence, methodically reduces synaptic connections. This isn't random clearing; it's a strategic process aimed at strengthening the most useful and frequently used neural pathways.

This careful pruning enhances the garden's overall function and beauty—it ensures plants have enough resources to thrive and that the garden remains tidy and functional. In the brain, this translates to improved efficiency in cognitive and emotional functioning. The remaining synaptic pathways after this pruning phase are faster and more efficient, much like how the well-pruned plants are healthier and more robust.

Understanding this transformative phase through the analogy of garden pruning not only illuminates the significance of these neurological changes but also highlights why this particular developmental stage is crucial for shaping a person's abilities and their way of interacting with the world. By maintaining the most effective pathways, the adolescent brain optimizes its operations much like a well-maintained garden offering a bountiful and beautiful yield.

Here is the detailed breakdown on the biochemical and cellular mechanisms involved in synaptic pruning during adolescence, a crucial process for brain development:

- **Cellular Mechanisms**:
  - **Neurons and Glial Cells**: Both neurons and glial cells, specifically microglia and astrocytes, play pivotal roles in synaptic pruning. Neurons continuously form and retract synaptic connections, while glial cells facilitate the removal of less active or weaker synapses.
  - **Apoptosis**: This process involves the programmed death of cells that are no longer needed, clearing the neural landscape for more efficient synaptic configurations.
  - **Phagocytosis**: Primarily conducted by microglia, this is the engulfing and digesting of cellular debris and weak synapses, which helps to refine neural circuits.
  - **Synaptic Tagging**: Neurons tag less active synapses with specific molecules, signaling microglia to target and prune these points of connection.

- **Biochemical Processes**:
  - **Key Molecules and Proteins**: Proteins such as C1q and MHC Class I molecules are instrumental in the identification and removal of synapses during pruning.
  - **Interaction with Neuronal Receptors**: C1q binds to receptors on neurons, tagging inefficient synapses for removal. Similarly, MHC-I molecules interact with receptors on microglia, guiding these immune cells to the sites of synaptic elimination.
  - **Mediation of Synaptic Strength and Elimination**: These interactions determine whether a synapse is strengthened or eliminated, based on the synaptic activity and necessity for efficient neural networking.

- **Regulation Factors**:

- **Neural Activity and Hormonal Changes**: Synaptic pruning is heavily regulated by the level of neural activity within brain circuits. Hormones released during adolescence, such as cortisol and sex hormones, also modulate synaptic pruning, reflecting the influence of both internal physiological factors and external stresses.

- **Impact of Environmental Influences**: Learning new skills or experiencing stress can accelerate synaptic pruning. For example, adolescents engaged in learning musical instruments or new languages may experience intensified synaptic refinement in relevant brain areas. Conversely, chronic stress can disrupt normal pruning processes, potentially leading to suboptimal neural development.

This comprehensive look into the specifics of synaptic pruning illuminates its complexity and necessity in adolescent brain development. Understanding these processes not only clarifies how the brain matures but also underscores the importance of nurturing environments that support healthy cognitive and emotional growth. By fostering conditions conducive to effective synaptic pruning, we can help ensure that adolescents develop robust neural networks that will serve them throughout life.

The adaptability of the brain, often referred to as plasticity, does not wane as we transition into adulthood or even later years; rather, it remains a pivotal aspect of our neurological framework, underpinning lifelong learning and cognitive flexibility. This continuous plasticity signifies that the adult brain is still capable of forming new neural connections in response to learning and experience.

In straightforward terms, adult brain plasticity involves the strengthening or weakening of synapses—the points of communication between neurons. This process is influenced by neuromodulators like dopamine, which enhances the brain's ability to encode new memories and skills, illustrating the brain's ongoing ability to adapt and remodel itself. For instance, consider the example of adults learning to play a musical instrument; this activity stimulates regions in the brain associated with auditory processing and motor control, effectively forging new pathways and strengthening existing ones.

Moreover, adult neurogenesis, particularly in the hippocampus, remains active and plays a critical role in how the brain adapts to new information and experiences. This ongoing generation of neurons is essential for processes like pattern separation, which is crucial for distinguishing between similar experiences and forming distinct memories.

Highlighting the real-world impact of this phenomenon, studies show that engaging in intellectually stimulating activities, such as learning new languages or challenging oneself with puzzles, can enhance and preserve cognitive functions in older adults. This is indicative of the brain's remarkable ability to not only maintain but also improve its functionality through continuous learning and engagement with diverse cognitive tasks.

Understanding the mechanisms of brain plasticity in adulthood and beyond not only deepens our comprehension of human biology but also empowers individuals to actively contribute to their cognitive health. By recognizing that the brain can adapt throughout one's life, supporting practices and lifestyles that encourage mental fitness becomes a clear path toward sustaining, and enhancing, cognitive capacities as we age. This knowledge shifts the narrative from inevitable decline to one of hopeful improvement, where each person has the potential to influence their cognitive vitality well into their later years.

Let's delve deeper into the molecular and cellular mechanisms that underscore the incredible capacity for plasticity in the adult brain.

Molecular Mechanisms:
- **Brain-Derived Neurotrophic Factor (BDNF)**: BDNF is a protein that plays a fundamental role in promoting synaptic plasticity by supporting the survival and growth of neurons. This neurotrophin facilitates the strengthening and formation of synapses, which are crucial for learning and memory.
    - **BDNF Signaling Pathways**: When BDNF binds to its receptor, TrkB, on neuron surfaces, it initiates a cascade of signaling events. These events include the activation of signaling proteins like AKT and mTOR, which ultimately lead to changes in gene expression and protein synthesis that strengthen synaptic connections and may lead to the growth of new synaptic connections.

Cellular Mechanisms:
- **Role of Glial Cells**:
    - **Astrocytes**: These star-shaped glial cells play a crucial

role in maintaining the chemical environment conducive to neural signaling. They regulate neurotransmitter levels by absorbing excess neurotransmitters from synaptic gaps and modulating synaptic strength and plasticity.

- **Oligodendrocytes and Myelination**: Oligodendrocytes generate myelin, the protective sheath that insulates neuronal axons, increasing the speed and efficiency of electrical signal transmission along neural pathways. Myelin plasticity, or changes in myelin thickness and configuration, can affect cognitive functions by altering conduction velocity and synchrony across neural networks.

Interplay Between Neurogenesis and Cognitive Functions:

- **Neurogenesis in the Hippocampus**: New neuron growth continues in the hippocampus, a region tied closely to memory formation and spatial navigation. These neurons integrate into existing circuits, where they contribute to forming and recalling memories.

- **Impact of Lifestyle Factors**: Regular physical exercise and cognitive engagement (like learning new skills or continuous education) have been shown to boost hippocampal neurogenesis. This activity suggests a reciprocal relationship where enhancing brain health through lifestyle choices further supports cognitive flexibility and learning in adulthood.

Understanding these mechanisms transforms our perception of adult brain capabilities. No longer seen as static, the adult brain is recognized for its dynamic potential to adapt continually—growing, learning, and reorganizing its neural architecture in response to ongoing experiences. This perspective not only enriches our understanding of the brain's complexity but also highlights the tremendous influence of our daily behaviors and environmental interactions on our cognitive health and capabilities as we age.

The Developing Brain expertly unravels the intricate process of brain development from infancy through adulthood, emphasizing the continuous and dynamic nature of neural plasticity and its significant implications for education, therapy, and general understanding of human growth. This comprehensive exploration reveals how the early years of life are critical due to heightened phases of synaptic formation and pruning, which significantly sculpt cognitive and emotional capacities. Such insights are crucial, illustrating why tailored early educational interventions can profoundly impact long-term developmental outcomes.

As adolescence ushers in further synaptic refinement, the text highlights the importance of supporting teenagers through environments that challenge and engage their evolving cognitive faculties. This stage is not just about physical growth but is pivotal in forming advanced reasoning and social skills.

Moreover, the discussion extends into adulthood, presenting compelling evidence that the brain retains its malleability; adults continue to forge new neural pathways in response to learning and experience. This plasticity ensures that adult learning and therapeutic strategies can be highly effective, promoting cognitive resilience and flexibility.

By detailing these processes, The Developing Brain underscores the lifelong potential for neurodevelopment and adaptation. This knowledge arms educators, therapists, and individuals with the understanding needed to foster environments that enhance cognitive and emotional well-being across the lifespan. It challenges the static view of the brain and replaces it with a model of continuous growth, advocating for ongoing intellectual engagement as a cornerstone of healthy brain development.

BRAIN DISORDERS AND DISEASES

Neurological disorders encompass a range of conditions that affect millions, from the cerebellum to neural pathways, with impacts that can deeply influence lives and societies. Take, for instance, the remarkable case of Stephen Hawking, a name synonymous not just with groundbreaking contributions to physics but also with his relentless battle with amyotrophic lateral sclerosis (ALS). Diagnosed at a young age, Hawking's experience with ALS illustrates the profound effects neurological diseases can have on a person's life, yet also how determination, technology, and medical support can combine to help manage the effects of such a formidable condition.

This chapter aims to pull back the curtain on the often-misunderstood realm of brain disorders and diseases, casting light on their symptoms, underlying causes, and the strides modern medicine has made in their treatment. As we explore these areas, the narrative will not just chart out the clinical facts but also delve into how these diseases alter daily lives, reshaping everything from routine tasks to interpersonal relationships. By understanding these impacts through real-world scenarios and scientific insights, the aim is not only to inform but also to foster a deeper empathy and comprehension of the trials and triumphs faced by those living with neurological disorders. This understanding is crucial not just for medical professionals and caregivers but for anyone eager to grasp the very real human experiences behind the medical terminology.

Neurological disorders, including Alzheimer's Disease, Parkinson's Disease, Epilepsy, and Multiple Sclerosis, each manifest through distinct pathophysiological processes that significantly affect bodily functions and quality of life. Understanding these disorders requires a clear grasp of their underlying mechanisms and clinical outcomes.

Alzheimer's Disease is characterized primarily by progressive memory loss and cognitive decline, stemming from neurodegeneration. This process involves the buildup of amyloid plaques and neurofibrillary tangles in the brain, which disrupt neural communication, eventually leading to neuronal death. The resultant symptoms often start subtly, like forgetting recent events, and gradually progress to more severe cognitive impairments.

Parkinson's Disease manifests through motor symptoms such as tremors, rigidity, and bradykinesia (slowed movement), largely due to the degeneration of dopamine-producing neurons in the substantia nigra, a critical area of the brain that regulates movement. This loss of dopamine creates a significant imbalance in neural signaling for motor control, often leading to the characteristic movements associated with the disorder.

Epilepsy, contrastingly, involves recurrent, unprovoked seizures, which are sudden surges of electrical activity in the brain. These can result from various causes, including genetic predispositions, brain injury, or developmental disorders. The manifestations of seizures can vary, ranging from brief lapses in attention or muscle jerks to severe and prolonged convulsions.

Multiple Sclerosis is noted for its attack on the body's own central nervous system, particularly the destruction of the myelin sheath that insulates nerve fibers. This demyelination leads to disrupted electrical signals throughout the brain and spinal cord, presenting in symptoms that can include visual disturbances, muscle weakness, and coordination problems.

These descriptions provide not just insight into what these diseases are but also why they affect individuals in such profound and varied ways. Each disorder disrupts the brain's normal functioning, yet they do so through unique mechanisms that require tailored approaches for management and treatment. Understanding these disorders down to their pathophysiological roots highlights the complexity of the brain and the pivotal importance of advancing our neurological and medical techniques to improve the lives of those affected.

Let's take a closer look at the molecular mechanisms that underpin Alzheimer's Disease, specifically focusing on how amyloid plaques and neurofibrillary tangles develop and their subsequent impact on neuronal communication.

Protein Misfolding and Aggregation:
Amyloid-beta proteins, normally soluble, can misfold under certain biochemical conditions, leading to aggregation. These misfolded proteins stick together, forming clumps that eventually become what we identify as amyloid plaques.

Factors such as genetic mutations, oxidative stress, and an imbalance in protein production and clearance can favor these processes. These plaques accumulate outside neurons and disrupt cell function by interfering with cell-to-cell signaling and increasing inflammatory responses, ultimately contributing to cell death.

Tau Protein Hyperphosphorylation:

Tau proteins play a crucial role in maintaining the stability of microtubules in nerve cells. In Alzheimer's Disease, abnormal chemical changes, specifically hyperphosphorylation of tau proteins, lead to the disintegration of these microtubules. Hyperphosphorylated tau proteins clump together to form tangles within neurons, which inhibit transport mechanisms essential for nutrient and information flow throughout the cell. This disruption can lead to neuronal malfunction and even cell death, exacerbating the cognitive decline seen in Alzheimer's patients.

Neuronal Communication Disruption:

The presence of amyloid plaques and tau tangles severely impairs neuronal communication. The plaques form a physical barrier that disrupts synaptic signaling, while the tangles distort the neuron's internal transport system, leading to synaptic loss and neuronal death. These disruptions in communication pathways are directly linked to the symptoms observed in Alzheimer's Disease, such as memory loss, cognitive decline, and changes in behavior.

Understanding these molecular details provides a clearer

picture of how Alzheimer's Disease manifests at a cellular level, explaining the progression from molecular dysfunction to the wide-ranging clinical symptoms seen in patients. This knowledge is crucial not only in developing therapeutic strategies that target these specific molecular derangements but also in devising preventive measures that might inhibit these processes before they lead to significant neurological damage. By grasping the complexities of these molecular interactions, one can appreciate the challenges involved in treating and researching Alzheimer's Disease, highlighting a continuous need for scientific exploration and innovation in this field.

Modern treatment approaches for neurological disorders integrate both traditional methods and cutting-edge technologies to manage and alleviate symptoms effectively. Among these, Deep Brain Stimulation (DBS) stands out, particularly in its application to conditions like Parkinson's Disease. DBS involves the surgical implantation of electrodes in specific areas of the brain, connected to a pulse generator implanted in the chest. This generator sends electrical impulses to the brain, helping to regulate abnormal impulses, or to affect certain cells and chemicals within the brain.

In the context of Parkinson's Disease, DBS is primarily targeted at the subthalamic nucleus or the globus pallidus, regions known to influence motor control. The stimulation can help reduce symptoms such as tremors, stiffness, and difficulty with walking, and may also reduce the need for medication by improving the overall motor function. The presence of the DBS system allows for adjustments in stimulation, making it a versatile tool adaptable to the patient's evolving condition.

The introduction of DBS showcases how intricately technology intersects with medical science, offering life-changing benefits for those with severe Parkinson's symptoms who do not respond well to traditional medications. It exemplifies a movement towards personalized medicine—an approach where treatments are tailored based on the individual's specific symptoms and responses.

However, as revolutionary as DBS and similar technologies are, they carry limitations and risks, including potential side effects like speech difficulties, muscle tightening, or unnatural movements, and the inherent risks associated with surgical procedures. Moreover, not all patients may be suitable candidates for such treatments, underscoring the importance of comprehensive patient evaluation and the need for ongoing advancements in technology and technique.

This exploration into modern treatments like DBS highlights not only the capabilities and sophistication of current medical practices but also the necessity for continuous research and development. By understanding both the potentials and the boundaries of these technologies, one gains a realistic appreciation for what can be achieved today and what might be possible tomorrow, emphasizing an ongoing commitment to improving life quality for individuals battling neurological disorders.

Deep Brain Stimulation (DBS) has emerged as a transformative treatment for Parkinson's Disease, especially beneficial for patients unresponsive to standard medication. Here's a detailed exploration of the DBS system, its implementation, and ongoing management.

<u>Detailed Components of DBS System</u>:
The DBS system primarily consists of three key components: the lead (electrode), the extension, and the pulse generator. The lead is a thin, insulated wire that ends in electrodes, placed strategically within specific brain regions. Commonly used electrodes are made from biocompatible materials like platinum-iridium, capable of delivering electrical impulses to brain tissue without corroding or degrading. The extension is another insulated wire that connects the lead to the pulse generator, a pacemaker-like device usually implanted under the skin in the chest. The pulse generator creates the electrical impulses controlled by programmable settings adjusted by medical professionals.

<u>Surgical Procedure of Implantation</u>:
The implantation of a DBS system involves multiple steps. Initially, a stereotactic head frame is fixed to the patient's head to stabilize and guide electrode placement via MRI or CT scans. Neurosurgeons then drill a small hole in the skull and insert the lead into the brain, targeting areas like the subthalamic nucleus or globus pallidus for Parkinson's Disease. Real-time feedback often guides the placement, ensuring optimal positioning. Once the electrodes are set, the extension wire is tunneled under the skin, connecting the lead to the pulse generator in the chest. Finally, the pulse

generator is programmed to the specific neurological needs of the patient.

Patient Selection Criteria:

Selecting the right candidates for DBS is crucial for treatment efficacy. Suitable patients typically have had Parkinson's Disease for at least five years and exhibit significant motor fluctuations or dyskinesias that are not optimally controlled by medication. Other key criteria include the absence of dementia or severe psychiatric conditions, as these can exacerbate treatment outcomes. Medical teams assess the overall health and neurological status to mitigate potential surgical risks or post-operative complications.

Adjustment and Management Post-Surgery:

Post-implantation, DBS requires careful adjustment to optimize the therapeutic outcomes. Neurologists adjust the settings on the pulse generator to fine-tune the frequency, amplitude, and duration of the electrical pulses, based on patient responses and symptom management needs. Follow-up appointments are crucial, especially in the initial months when medication adjustments are also likely. Long-term management involves regular check-ups to reassess the system's settings, battery replacements every few years, and ongoing assessment of neurological and physical health.

Understanding these facets of Deep Brain Stimulation provides insights into the precise and complex nature of treating neurological disorders like Parkinson's Disease. This clarity not only informs potential candidates and their families but also ensures that healthcare providers can better strategize and tailor treatment plans for effective management and improved patient outcomes.

Imagine going about your day with the unpredictability of a rapidly changing weather system inside you. For individuals living with neurological disorders, each day can feel just like navigating an internal climate that shifts without warning. One moment the sun is shining—symptoms are manageable, and activities feel attainable. Suddenly, a storm brews; tremors, memory lapses, or muscle stiffness set in, much like a sudden downpour that forces you to alter your path or cancel plans.

This fluctuating internal weather makes simple tasks like buttoning a shirt or recalling a well-known address daunting, not just occasionally, but possibly multiple times within a single day. The societal impact of these conditions extends beyond the individual. It involves family, friends, and even broader societal structures like workplaces and public spaces, all of which must adapt to the varying needs of individuals affected by these unpredictable internal storms.

Just as cities and communities might prepare for erratic weather through early warnings and adaptable infrastructure, a greater societal understanding and accommodation for neurological disorders are crucial. It's not just about making physical spaces accessible but also about fostering an environment where the unpredictable nature of these conditions is acknowledged and planned for, allowing individuals to navigate their days with dignity and safety, despite the unpredictable weather within. This analogy helps us grasp the daily reality for those with neurological disorders and underscores the importance of supportive structures that respond to their ever-changing needs.

Here is the breakdown on societal accommodations needed for individuals with neurological disorders, ensuring inclusivity and support across various environments:

- **Public Infrastructure**:
    - **Transportation**: Public transport systems can incorporate features such as low-floor buses for easier boarding, dedicated spaces for wheelchairs, and visual as well as auditory announcements to aid those with sensory impairments.
    - **Buildings**: Doors with automatic openers, elevators with auditory signals, and ramps where stairs might be a barrier are essential modifications. Visual guides or maps should be clear and simple to follow for those with cognitive challenges.
    - **Parks and Public Spaces**: Paths with tactile paving to guide individuals with visual impairments, shaded seating areas for those sensitive to overstimulation, and clear signage are fundamental. Emergency services within these spaces should also be readily accessible with instructions that are easy to understand.

- **Workplace Adjustments**:
    - **Flexible Work Hours**: Allowing employees with neurological disorders to have flexible working hours can accommodate varying energy levels and symptom severity throughout the day.
    - **Quiet Rooms**: Providing spaces where individuals can

retreat when overwhelmed or in need of rest can be crucial for managing symptoms like anxiety or sensory overload.

 - **Customized Workstations**: Ergonomic adjustments in the workspace, such as adjustable desks, chairs with proper support, and customized lighting, can significantly reduce physical strain and boost productivity.

 - **Social Support Systems**:
 - **Community Support Groups**: Facilitating platforms where individuals can share experiences, offer mutual support, and learn from others facing similar challenges fosters a strong sense of community and belonging.
 - **Counseling Services**: Accessible mental health services that specialize in neurological disorders can help individuals navigate their conditions and deal with the psychological impact, enhancing overall well-being.
 - **Educational Programs**: Informing families and caregivers about neurological disorders through workshops or seminars can empower them with the knowledge to provide better care and support.

This detailed outline emphasizes that taking these steps not only assists individuals directly affected by neurological disorders but also educates and informs the wider community, promoting a society that values accessibility and inclusion. By understanding and implementing these measures, communities can ensure that everyone, regardless of neurological condition, can participate fully and with dignity in all aspects of life.

Treating brain disorders, particularly Alzheimer's disease, presents a labyrinth of complexities that challenge both therapeutic management and patient care. Alzheimer's disease, driven by the intricate interplay of genetic, environmental, and lifestyle factors, manifests as a gradual decline in cognitive function, fundamentally altering an individual's ability to remember, think, and reason.

The core challenge in treating Alzheimer's lies in its elusive etiology. Despite extensive research, the precise causes remain only partially understood. This disease involves the accumulation of amyloid plaques and tau tangles in the brain, which disrupt neuronal communication. The complexity escalates because these pathological changes can begin decades before the appearance of clinical symptoms, complicating early detection and intervention.

Another formidable hurdle is the current lack of a cure. Existing treatments primarily focus on symptom management rather than addressing the disease's progression. Medications such as cholinesterase inhibitors and memantine can help manage cognitive symptoms, but their efficacy varies and diminishes as the disease progresses. This limitation underscores the need for a multi-faceted treatment approach that includes medical, psychological, and social care to support the comprehensive needs of patients.

From a care perspective, the progressive nature of Alzheimer's necessitates increasingly intensive care arrangements. This progression can place a substantial emotional and financial strain on families and caregivers, highlighting the necessity for robust support systems and resources. As patients lose their ability to perform everyday tasks, the responsibility on caregivers grows, requiring not just physical care but also profound patience and understanding.

In conclusion, the treatment of Alzheimer's disease demands not only medical innovation to unravel and target its complex pathophysiology but also a compassionate framework for patient care. Each step forward in understanding and treating Alzheimer's not only illuminates the intricate workings of the human brain but also enhances our capacity to extend care and improve life quality for those affected, marking profound implications for future advancements in neurodegenerative disease management.

Let's take a deeper look at the molecular pathology of Alzheimer's disease, focusing on how amyloid plaques and tau tangles contribute to neuronal dysfunction.

<u>Biochemical Formation of Amyloid Plaques</u>:
In Alzheimer's disease, the processing of amyloid precursor proteins (APP) is crucially altered. Normally, APP is split by enzymes in a way that prevents any harmful byproducts. However, in Alzheimer's, abnormal enzymatic activities, particularly by beta-secretase and gamma-secretase, lead to the production of beta-amyloid fragments. These sticky fragments accumulate to form amyloid plaques. These plaques deposit between neurons, disrupting cell function by interfering with neuron-to-neuron communication at synapses and initiating inflammatory processes that can lead to cell death.

Tau Protein Phosphorylation and Tangle Formation:

Tau proteins are integral to maintaining the stability of microtubules in neuronal cells, which are essential for nutrient transport and cellular structure. In Alzheimer's disease, abnormal chemical changes cause the hyperphosphorylation of tau proteins, which means adding too many phosphate groups to tau proteins. This excess phosphorylation causes tau to detach from microtubules, leading them to collapse and form tangled, twisted strands within neuron axons. These tangles block the neuron's transport system, which can cause the nerve cell to die.

Impact on Neuronal Communication:

The presence of amyloid plaques and tau tangles severely impairs the ability of neurons to communicate. This disruption is due to the interference in the synaptic activity where nerve cells communicate. The plaques and tangles can distort signal transmission, leading to memory lapses, language problems, and other cognitive declines typical of Alzheimer's disease. These molecular changes manifest as the symptoms commonly observed in patients, such as disorientation and mood swings, bridging the gap between cellular pathology and clinical presentation.

Understanding these molecular and cellular processes elucidates why Alzheimer's disease is so challenging to treat. Each step in the degeneration process—from protein misfolding to the breakdown of neuronal communication—reveals potential targets for treatment but also highlights the complexity of reversing or preventing these changes. By grasively tackling these scientific concepts, we not only deepen our comprehension of the disease but also enhance our capacity to support those affected in more scientifically informed and empathetic ways.

The future of neurological research holds promising advancements in gene therapy and personalized medicine, potentially revolutionizing treatment approaches for patients with brain disorders. Gene therapy, targeting the fundamental genetic abnormalities causing neurological diseases, offers a profound shift from symptomatic treatment to potentially curative interventions. For conditions like Huntington's disease or certain forms of Alzheimer's linked to specific genetic mutations, introducing correct genetic material into a patient's cells could directly address the root causes of these disorders.

Personalized medicine, fueled by advancements in genomics and biotechnology, tailors treatments to individual patients based on their genetic profile and specific disease characteristics. This approach not only promises enhanced efficacy but also aims to reduce adverse effects by aligning therapies closely with each patient's unique biological context. An example of this is the use of biomarkers in Alzheimer's disease to identify the stage of the disease and tailor interventions accordingly, potentially slowing or halting disease progression much more effectively than current standard care.

Navigating the complexities of the human brain requires an ever-evolving understanding of its mechanisms. Both gene therapy and personalized medicine stand out as beacons of hope, offering new pathways that could lead to substantial improvements in the lives of individuals facing debilitating brain disorders. As we advance these technologies, the potential to convert profound medical insights into practical, life-altering treatments grows, marking a significant shift towards more targeted and effective management of neurological conditions.

Through the intricate exploration of brain disorders and diseases, we've navigated the complex web of pathologies, treatments, and the human stories intertwined with these conditions. Advancements in medical science, including groundbreaking research in genetics, neuroimaging, and pharmacology, continually push the boundaries of what we can achieve in diagnosing and managing these conditions. Each discovery not only enhances our scientific understanding but also improves the precision and effectiveness of treatments, opening new doors to therapeutic possibilities that were once considered unattainable.

Simultaneously, growing public awareness plays a crucial role in shaping the narratives of individuals affected by neurological disorders. As society gains a deeper understanding and empathy towards these conditions, the stigma often associated with such diagnoses diminishes. This cultural shift is pivotal, fostering an environment where individuals feel supported and empowered to seek help and share their experiences.

This journey through the landscape of brain disorders reaffirms the power of medical innovation and societal understanding to transform lives. The collaboration between researchers, healthcare professionals, patients, and the public is essential in crafting a future where every individual facing neurological challenges can access the support and treatment they need to lead fulfilling lives. While the path forward may present new challenges, the unyielding pursuit of knowledge and compassion ensures that our collective efforts will continue to make significant positive impacts on the lives of many.

THE FUTURE OF BRAIN RESEARCH

The frontier of brain research stands as one of the most exhilarating aspects of modern science, poised to unfold mysteries that have puzzled humanity for centuries. Today, the rapid evolution of technologies and methodologies offers unprecedented opportunities to not only explore but potentially revolutionize our understanding of the human brain. Emerging tools like neuroimaging, gene editing, and artificial intelligence are reshaping what we thought possible, turning science fiction into science reality. These advancements hold the promise to unlock the intricate workings of neurological functions and pave the way for innovative treatments for brain disorders, potentially altering the course of medicine and how we perceive human cognition and mental health. As we venture into this exploration, this chapter aims to guide you through these complex concepts with clarity and precision, offering insights into how each new tool and technique could fundamentally transform our approach to neurological health. Through this journey, our objective is to provide you with a clear, comprehensive understanding of the seismic shifts occurring in brain research, all while maintaining an engaging and approachable dialogue. Let's uncover the layers of this dynamic field together, examining not just the mechanics, but the profound implications each breakthrough holds for the future.

Neuroinformatics stands at the intersection of neuroscience and information technology, harnessing vast data to unravel the complexities of brain activity. This advanced field employs powerful computational tools and algorithms to analyze and synthesize neurological data collected from diverse sources such as MRI scans, EEGs, and molecular genetics. Imagine a situation where millions of data points from brain scans are like individual stars in the night sky. Neuroinformatics uses these stars to map constellations; in this context, it maps patterns and connections within the brain.

For example, when studying cognitive functions such as memory or learning, neuroinformatics tools can identify specific patterns of neural activity triggered during these processes. These patterns, once opaque due to the sheer volume and complexity of the data, become clearer through sophisticated models that can simulate brain processes. The technology acts much like a translator or decoder, transforming raw, often chaotic neurological signals into organized, understandable maps of brain activity.

This transformation is crucial, as it allows researchers and clinicians to visualize and understand the functional areas of the brain in ways that were not possible before. It answers fundamental questions about which parts of the brain are involved in certain activities, how different areas of the brain communicate, and how this communication can be disrupted in the case of neurological diseases.

By providing a detailed view of the brain's intricate workings, neuroinformatics not only advances the scientific understanding of the brain but also enhances the development of targeted therapies for disorders like Alzheimer's or Parkinson's disease. The potential of neuroinformatics extends to improving diagnostic accuracy and tailoring personalized treatment plans that address the specific needs of patients based on their unique brain activity patterns.

Thus, neuroinformatics is not just about data collection and analysis; it is about paving a clearer path to understanding the most complex organ in the human body and solving some of the most persistent puzzles of medical science. With each advancement in this field, the prospects for better patient outcomes and more effective treatments become increasingly tangible.

In neuroinformatics, the journey from acquiring brain data to developing therapeutic applications involves several meticulous steps:

Data Collection: Neuroinformatics integrates diverse types of brain data. Electroencephalograms (EEGs) capture electrical activities showing brain wave patterns. Functional magnetic resonance imaging (fMRI) provides insight into brain areas activated during tasks by measuring changes in blood flow, indicating mental engage level. Genomic data links biological markers with brain functions to understand genetic influences on neurobehavioral traits. Collecting this varied data allows researchers to paint a detailed picture of brain structure and activity under numerous conditions.

Data Processing: Before any meaningful analysis, raw data must be refined and standardized. This preprocessing includes normalization, which adjusts values to a common scale, and noise reduction to remove irrelevant or random data disturbances, enhancing signal clarity. Data alignment ensures that observations from different datasets correspond to the same temporal or spatial points, crucial when combining multiple data types or sources.

Pattern Recognition: Once processed, the data is analyzed to identify meaningful patterns or anomalies. Machine learning techniques are employed, where algorithms learn from data to identify and predict trends without being explicitly programmed. Neural networks, which mimic human brain operations, are particularly effective in recognizing complex patterns from large datasets. These tools categorize data based on learned characteristics, revealing hidden insights about brain functions and dysfunctions.

Simulation and Modeling: Identified patterns are used to simulate brain activities or model neurological conditions. Software tools like MATLAB or Python libraries such as TensorFlow support these activities, allowing researchers to construct models that mimic real-world brain behavior or test hypotheses about neurological responses. These simulations help in visualizing how certain diseases might evolve within the brain and what factors influence these changes.

Application in Therapy Development: Models and

simulations inform therapy developments, guiding interventions to be both effective and personalized. By predicting disease trajectories or assessing how different therapeutic strategies might alter disease progression, researchers can design targeted treatments. For example, a model predicting the advancement of Alzheimer's based on early-pattern recognition can help in formulating early intervention strategies that slow the disease's progression, radically tailoring patient care.

By harnessing advanced computational processes, neuroinformatics not only deepens our understanding of brain complexities but also enhances the potential for significant therapeutical advances, the effects of which resonate profoundly across neuroscience and patient care. Each step in this chain from data collection to therapeutic development builds upon the last to create a comprehensive framework that could potentially transform neurological healthcare.

Imagine you're a skilled craftsman, and your task is to restore an exquisite, ancient clock. This clock, however, isn't just any ordinary clock but represents the complex genetic makeup of the human brain. In gene therapy for brain disorders, scientists work much like master craftsmen with a molecular toolkit. Each tool in this kit is precisely designed for specific tasks — to tweak, repair, or replace parts of the molecular machinery within our cells, which analogous to the gears and springs in the clock.

This molecular toolkit is equipped with various innovative instruments, one of which includes CRISPR-Cas9, a groundbreaking technology that functions like a pair of microscopic scissors. These scissors can cut DNA at exact locations, allowing scientists to remove faulty segments (similar to removing a rusted gear) and replace them with healthy ones, essentially correcting errors right at the source. It's similar to finding the precise gear that causes the clock to malfunction and substituting it with one that ensures smooth operation.

Apart from CRISPR, other tools like zinc finger nucleases and TALENs operate on similar principles but differ slightly in how they identify the DNA segments they need to correct. Think of them as different types of screwdrivers, each tailored for specific screws in the mechanism.

The potential of these tools is vast. They offer hope in addressing genetic disorders like Huntington's or certain forms of inherited Alzheimer's by directly fixing the genetic abnormalities that cause these conditions. It's much like repairing the clock's faulty mechanism that causes it to lose time, thereby restoring its functionality and prolonging its lifespan.

Using gene therapy to correct gene mutations is like performing meticulous repairs on our genetic clockwork, demonstrating how this advanced approach has profound implications not only for treating diseases but also in understanding the intricate workings of the human brain. This blend of genetics and therapy illuminates a path towards a future where many brain disorders could be managed more effectively, ensuring better health outcomes and quality of life. Thus, the analogy of a molecular toolkit not only simplifies the concept of gene therapy but also highlights its transformative potential in neuroscientific research and medicine.

Here is the detailed breakdown of the gene editing process used in therapies for brain disorders:

- **Target Identification**:
    - **Gene Sequencing**: Scientists utilize advanced sequencing technologies to read the genetic codes, allowing them to identify mutations or irregularities linked to neurological disorders.
    - **Genomic Mapping**: Techniques like whole-genome mapping provide a comprehensive view of an individual's genetic landscape, pinpointing specific areas of interest that may contribute to brain disorders.

- **Gene Editing Tools**:
    - **CRISPR-Cas9**: This tool uses a guide RNA to identify the exact DNA sequence that needs editing and employs the Cas9 protein to create a break at that specific location in the DNA strand.
        - **Mechanism of Action**: The guide RNA is designed to match the DNA sequence of the target gene. Once bound, Cas9 cuts the DNA, allowing scientists to remove or add nucleotides to correct genetic errors.
    - **Zinc Finger Nucleases (ZFNs)**: These are proteins engineered to bind to specific DNA sequences and introduce cuts, which can then be used to insert or delete genetic material.
        - **Mechanism of Action**: ZFNs use a zinc finger

protein to recognize the target DNA sequence and a FokI nuclease domain to cut the DNA precisely at the targeted location.

- **TALENs (Transcription Activator-Like Effector Nucleases)**: Similar to ZFNs but use different DNA-binding domains to enhance targeting precision.
   - **Mechanism of Action**: TALENs leverage transcription activator-like effectors that bind to specific DNA bases, linked to a nuclease that cuts the DNA.

- **Delivery Systems**:
   - **Viral Vectors**: Commonly used to deliver gene-editing tools into cells due to their natural ability to enter cells and deliver genetic material.
      - **Adeno-Associated Viruses (AAVs)**: Widely used due to their lower pathogenicity and ability to target different types of cells, including neurons.
   - **Nanoparticle-Based Delivery**: Offers a non-viral approach, using nanoparticles to encapsulate and protect gene-editing enzymes until they reach their target cells in the brain.
      - **Mechanism**: Nanoparticles are designed to cross the blood-brain barrier and release their cargo directly into brain cells, minimizing systemic exposure.

- **Outcome Assessment**:
   - **Neuroimaging**: Techniques such as MRI and PET scans are employed to observe changes in brain structure and function after treatment.
   - **Biomarkers**: Blood or cerebrospinal fluid is analyzed for molecular indicators that reflect genetic corrections at the cellular level or signs of improvement in brain function.

- **Application**: These biomarkers help measure the efficacy of the gene therapy and monitor any long-term effects or potential side effects.

This comprehensive guide highlights the step-by-step approach in utilizing gene therapy techniques for treating brain disorders, emphasizing the precision and innovative strategies that are at the forefront of neuroscience.

Studying human consciousness is similar to deciphering a highly sophisticated computer code that orchestrates the operations of an advanced robot. Just as a robot operates based on the intricacies of its programmed code, human consciousness emerges from the complex interactions within the brain's vast network of neurons.

To start, consider the robot's code as a blueprint that dictates every action, reaction, and interaction the machine undertakes. In a similar manner, the human brain functions on an intricate web of neural circuits, each firing electrical impulses and releasing chemicals to communicate. This neural activity forms the basis of thoughts, emotions, and behaviors—components of what we understand as consciousness.

Deciphering this 'code' within the brain involves mapping out billions of neural connections and understanding how these connections produce conscious experience. This process can be thought of as trying to understand every line of code in a system as complex as artificial intelligence—where altering one line can change the machine's behavior.

Researchers use various methods such as brain imaging and electrophysiological studies to trace these neural pathways and observe how they respond to different stimuli.

However, much like debugging a complex algorithm, exploring consciousness challenges scientists to not only map these connections but also to comprehend how they synchronize to manifest coherent and intentional behaviors. The execution must be flawless; any misstep in interpretation can lead to misconceptions about how consciousness forms.

The effort to unravel this mystery is continuous, with new technologies and methodologies shedding light on previously opaque aspects of neural function. Still, the challenge persists, similar to software engineers perpetually upgrading and refining AI to mimic human-like awareness and decision-making more closely.

Thus, the study of consciousness is not only about mapping out neural connections or observing brain activity. It is about piecing together these observations to form a cohesive understanding of how subjective experiences and perceptions of the world arise—much like assembling a myriad of code into a seamless, functioning software. This ongoing exploration not only deepens our understanding of the human mind but also bridges the gap between biological neural networks and artificial intelligence.

Let's take a deeper look at the methodologies utilized in studying consciousness through various brain imaging and electrophysiological techniques, detailing their specific contributions to our understanding of neural activities associated with conscious experience.

Types of Brain Imaging:
- **Functional Magnetic Resonance Imaging (fMRI)**: fMRI is instrumental in tracking changes in blood flow related to neural activity in the brain. When a specific brain region is more active, it consumes more oxygen, and fMRI detects these areas by monitoring changes in blood oxygen levels. This allows scientists to observe which parts of the brain are involved during different tasks or states of consciousness.
- **Positron Emission Tomography (PET)**: PET imaging involves injecting a radioactive tracer into the bloodstream, which helps to highlight active areas of the brain based on glucose consumption. This method is particularly useful for exploring the brain's metabolic processes and how they relate to conscious thought and cognition.
- **Electroencephalography (EEG)**: EEG records electrical activity directly from the scalp. The technique captures fluctuations in voltage resulting from ionic current flows within the neurons of the brain, offering real-time data on brain wave patterns. This is crucial for studying the temporal dynamics of consciousness and understanding how fast the brain responds to stimuli.

Electrophysiological Techniques:
- **Single Neuron Recording**: This technique involves placing electrodes near individual neurons to record their electrical activity. By measuring the action potentials or spikes from single neurons, researchers can infer how

specific cells contribute to different conscious experiences.

- **Patch Clamping**: Patch clamping allows detailed study of ionic currents in individual neurons by attaching a tiny glass pipette to a small patch of neuronal membrane. This method helps in understanding how single neurons process signals which contribute to higher cognitive functions, including consciousness.

The information collected from these recordings is analyzed to map how neurons within a network interact, and how these interactions correlate with different states of consciousness.

Data Analysis in Consciousness Studies:
- **Computational Models**: Advanced computational techniques integrate data from fMRI, PET, EEG, and neuron-specific recordings to create models that simulate brain activity. These models help hypothesize how different neural networks support various aspects of consciousness.
- **Data Synthesis**: The integration of multi-modal imaging data facilitates a more comprehensive understanding of how various brain regions contribute to the formation of conscious experience. Sophisticated software tools analyze these large datasets to discern patterns, allowing researchers to hypothesize about the neural correlates of consciousness.

Through these methodologies, the landscape of consciousness research becomes clearer and more accessible. Each tool and technique offers a unique lens through which the complex architecture and dynamics of the brain are interpreted and understood. As these methods evolve, they continue to refine our understanding of the most enigmatic aspects of human cognition, providing invaluable insights into the very essence of human thought and awareness.

Emerging technologies that modify brain activity present a significant advance in medical science, yet they also bring forth a complex array of ethical considerations. As we stand on the brink of capabilities that could radically alter human cognition and behavior, it becomes crucial to assess the balance between innovative treatment potentials and the moral responsibilities they entail.

Modifying brain activity can offer unprecedented benefits, such as reversing the debilitating effects of neurological diseases or enhancing cognitive functions, which could improve quality of life significantly. However, these technologies also raise serious ethical questions about consent, privacy, and the potential for misuse. For instance, who decides which aspects of behavior or cognition are desirable for enhancement? What are the implications of having technologies that can potentially access or alter a person's thoughts without their full, informed consent?

Another pivotal concern is the long-term impact of brain activity modification. While initial outcomes might seem beneficial, there is a profound need for studies that explore long-term effects, which remain largely unknown. This uncertainty requires a cautious approach, integrating rigorous clinical trials and ethical oversight to ensure that the benefits unequivocally outweigh the risks.

Furthermore, there is the issue of accessibility and fairness. Advanced neurotechnologies could exacerbate social inequalities if only a segment of the population can afford them. It is imperative to consider how these technologies are deployed in society to prevent scenarios where only the wealthy benefit from enhancements or treatments.

In discussing the ethics of modifying brain activity, it becomes clear that while the scientific potential is vast, the ethical landscape is equally extensive and complex. This discourse necessitates ongoing, transparent dialogues among scientists, ethicists, policymakers, and the public to navigate these uncharted waters responsibly. Only through collective, well-informed decision-making can we harness the full potential of these technologies while upholding the fundamental values of human dignity and equality.

Let's take a deeper look at the ethical frameworks used to govern the use of brain-modifying technologies, diving into the specific mechanisms and measures that ensure these advancements are managed responsibly.

Ethical Guidelines and Principles:
- Neurotechnologies, like any other medical technology, are governed by a set of ethical guidelines that ensure research and applications are conducted responsibly. Researchers and clinicians are expected to adhere to principles such as beneficence, non-maleficence, autonomy, and justice.
    - **Institutional Review Boards (IRB) and Ethical**

Committees: These bodies play a crucial role by reviewing research proposals to make sure they meet ethical standards before any study is conducted. They assess the potential risks versus the benefits, ensure that all data privacy laws are adhered to, and that participant welfare is protected.

Consent Processes:
- Obtaining informed consent is paramount in neurotechnology trials to ensure that participants are fully aware of what the research involves, including any potential risks and benefits.
- **Communicating Risks**: Participants are clearly informed about the procedures, the nature of the technology used, potential risks, and consequences. Special attention is given to how information is presented to ensure it is understandable. For individuals with cognitive impairments, researchers ensure that consent is obtained through legally authorized representatives and that these participants can comprehend the information to the extent possible.

Equity and Accessibility:
- Ensuring that these advanced technologies are accessible across different socio-economic groups is a significant concern. Strategies implemented include policy-making aimed at regulating costs and distribution of these technologies.
- **Subsidies and Regulation**: Various initiatives may include government subsidies for neurotechnological treatments and regulations that require insurance companies to cover these interventions, aiming to prevent a scenario where only the affluent benefit from high-tech treatments.

Long-term Surveillance:
- Monitoring the effects of brain-modifying technologies over the long term is crucial to identify any delayed adverse effects and to verify the sustained effectiveness of the treatments.

- **Ongoing Assessments**: These are carried out using follow-up visits, continuous remote monitoring through wearable devices, and periodic reassessments using the same or similar diagnostic tools used in the initial treatment phase. This proactive surveillance helps in tweaking treatments as necessary and in providing real-time data on patient progress.

Through this meticulous approach integrating ethical, legal, and clinical perspectives, the use of brain-modifying technologies is conducted with a heightened sense of responsibility to participants and society. Such comprehensive management ensures ethical dilemmas are navigated with informed consent, and the benefits of neurotechnological advances are distributed justly and safely.

Advances in brain research hold transformative potential for addressing neurological conditions that affect millions worldwide. By diving deeper into the complexities of the brain, scientists are not only deciphering the underlying mechanisms of disorders but also paving the way for revolutionary treatments that could dramatically enhance patient outcomes.

Through sophisticated imaging techniques and molecular genetics, researchers can now observe the brain's activity in real-time and at an unprecedented level of detail. This ability to monitor neural interactions and changes at the molecular level contributes significantly to our understanding of diseases like Alzheimer's, Parkinson's, and epilepsy. As a result, the prospect of personalized medicine becomes increasingly tangible, where treatments can be tailored to the specific genetic makeup and disease progression in individual patients.

Moreover, ongoing developments in neurotechnology, such as brain-computer interfaces, offer hope for restoring function and improving life quality for those with traumatic brain injuries or stroke. These technologies could enable individuals to regain mobility and communication skills, substantially reducing the long-term disabilities associated with severe neurological damage.

The expansion of knowledge in brain science is not just about creating better medical interventions; it's about offering a renewed sense of hope and possibility for patients and their families. As we continue to uncover more about how the brain works, the potential to overcome present and future challenges becomes not just an aspiration but a foreseeable reality. This journey into the brain's deepest workings underscores a growing optimism that many of the most daunting neurological puzzles can, and will, be solved.

CONCLUSION

As we close the final pages of "The Brain Explained," it's worth pausing to reflect on the fascinating journey through the complexities and marvels of the human brain. From the intricate dance of neurons firing in our cerebral cortex to the deep mysteries of consciousness, this book has aimed to illuminate the labyrinth of our minds with clarity and simplicity. Through vivid examples and relatable analogies, we've explored the different sections and functions of the brain, making advanced concepts accessible and engaging.

Throughout the book, several key themes have emerged: the brain's incredible adaptability, its fundamental role in shaping our identity and experiences, and the profound implications of neurological research on everyday life. We've learned that the brain is not just an isolated organ but a dynamic, interconnected system that influences and is influenced by every aspect of our being.

One of the most crucial lessons is the concept of neuroplasticity – the brain's ability to change and adapt throughout our lives. This understanding underscores the potential for recovery and growth, even in the face of neurological challenges. It also carries a message of hope for those affected by brain injuries or disorders, highlighting the brain's inherent capacity to find new pathways and create new connections.

The discussions on how lifestyle, environment, and technology affect our neural wiring have perhaps raised more questions than answers, inviting us to consider how our choices and surroundings shape our cognitive functions and mental health. This dialogue between neuroscience and daily life encourages a proactive approach to not only understanding but also nurturing our brain health.

As you set this book aside, may you carry forward a deeper appreciation for the intricate organ that resides within your skull. May the knowledge that every thought, emotion, and memory involves a symphony of neural activity inspire you to think differently about your mental habits and health. The journey of understanding the brain is far from complete – it is a rapidly evolving field, and each discovery opens new doors to understanding what makes us uniquely human.

In conclusion, "The Brain Explained" serves not just as a guidebook to the brain but as an invitation to continue exploring, questioning, and marveling at one of nature's most extraordinary creations. Here's to the ongoing journey of discovery, to the mysteries that remain unsolved, and to the continuous quest for knowledge that pushes the boundaries of what we know about the magical, mysterious brain.

ABOUT THE AUTHOR

Alex Rossi brings a wealth of experience from over twenty years in the information technology industry, having worked with some of the world's leading tech giants.

With a deep-seated passion for science, technology, and languages, Alex excels at demystifying complex subjects, making them accessible and engaging to a broad audience. His writings focus on breaking down intricate topics into everyday terms, helping readers not just learn but also apply this knowledge in their daily lives.

Currently, Alex is a proud member of Green Mountain Publishing, which publishes his insightful books. Through his work, he aims to foster a deeper understanding and appreciation of technology and science, enriching readers' lives.

Printed in Great Britain
by Amazon